(Un)covering Men

First published by Fanele – an imprint of Jacana Media (Pty) Ltd – in 2012
10 Orange Street
Sunnyside
Auckland Park 2092
South Africa
+2711 628 3200
www.jacana.co.za

© Anova Health Institute, Wits Journalism Programme and individual contributors, 2012
HIV & AIDS Media Project
Anova Health Institute and Wits Journalism Programme
12 Sherborne Road
Parktown 2193
(+27 11) 715 5800
www.journaids.org
@HIVandtheMedia

This publication is made possible by the US President's Emergency Plan for AIDS Relief
(PEPFAR) through the United States Agency for International Development (USAID),
under the terms of the award Cooperative Agreement No. 674-00-08-00039-00
administered by Johns Hopkins Health and Education in South Africa (JHHESA) and the
Anova Health Institute. The opinions expressed herein are those of the authors
and do not necessarily reflect the views of USAID or PEPFAR.

ISBN 978-1-920196-58-5

Design and layout by Geraldine Hendler / squareart
Cover design by publicide
Spine image: Frik Myburgh, Gugulethu
Set in Warnock Pro Light 10.5/15
Printed by Ultra Litho (Pty) Ltd, Johannesburg
Job no. 1825

See a complete list of Jacana titles at www.jacana.co.za

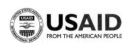 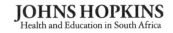

(Un)covering Men

Rewriting Masculinity & Health
in South Africa

edited by
Melissa Meyer & Helen Struthers

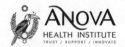 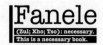

Contents

Photographic essays

The world recently commemorated the 30th anniversary since the first case of HIV was reported. A lot has happened since then – good and bad. The positive achievements made in the response to HIV give us something to celebrate. But at the same time there is still a lot of work to be done.

Many people are still getting infected with HIV, many are still dying and many more are still suffering the consequences of stigma and discrimination. And this is why the timing of this book is very important.

In 1999, when I found out that I had HIV, there were less than 2 million people living with the virus in South Africa. Before my own diagnosis, I had never met a person who was HIV positive. Today there are nearly 6 million – and close to half of those are men.

Back then I found the issues the media reported to be quite alarming. I remember a headline splashed across national newspapers, just a few months before I tested positive: Gugu Dlamini from KwaZulu-Natal was killed for disclosing her HIV status.

Soon after I learned about my status, another headline read: "HIV to be made a notifiable disease". It scared me. I was not ready for anyone to know about my status. Like me, that news made many people living with HIV recoil from public spaces. While I was trying to get over the initial shock, the country entered an era of AIDS denialism. That did little to help my situation.

The media became a platform for debate between those who acknowledged the existence of HIV and those who denied it. These discussions left many South Africans confused about their role in the epidemic.

Another milestone around that time was the campaign for a successful implementation of prevention of mother-to-child transmission (PMTCT). It placed a significant amount of focus on affected women and their babies, which of course was a good thing. But men were glaringly absent – and that was reflected in media coverage.

As a result, we had a society split into two when it came to HIV – those who believed HIV was not their problem and those who were affected. Often that split drew a harsh line between men and women.

It puzzles me that in my 14th year of living with HIV we are still talking about the need to involve men in both HIV programmes and media coverage. This is despite "renewed energy" by politicians in the fight against HIV. I expected that by now this would have changed, and that the change would be reflected in HIV reporting that is balanced and more consistent.

Yet coupled with recent careless coverage of antiretroviral side-effects, I can't help but conclude that much of our current HIV news has been reduced to sensation; when what we really need are stories that will engage positively with everyone (men included) on our roles in this bid for our lives.

Campaigns like *Brothers for Life* and Soul City's television programmes are playing their part in placing emphasis on men's roles, but we have a long road to go.

I asked my friend Nelo, who is also living with HIV, what her views are about men and the epidemic. Her response was frank: "Men aren't hiding. We just live in a country where men are immune to the virus. They are 'fine'. They are 'OK'. HIV has nothing to do with them. And all the women in South Africa are probably getting the virus from the water they drink."

Nelo has a point. But I can't help but wonder about the experiences that drove her to these conclusions.

For the past 13 years, I have been living publicly with HIV, and through my work I have been helping others open up about their status. My journey has shown me how different men can be and how these differences show in their responses to HIV: from men who refuse to acknowledge their role when an HIV infection comes to their home, to men who are doing exceptional work educating their peers and supporting their partners at home.

This book is coming out at a time when South Africa desperately needs consistent and positive reporting that engages men – especially when it comes to communicating the role men can, and must, play in the response to HIV. Like Nelo said, we must continue to challenge false perceptions and cultural myths that create an impression that "HIV has nothing to do with men".

From my own experience I know that men can have a positive impact, not just on the epidemic, but on the lives of their families and communities.

Now I would like to read about *that* in the news.

Pholokgolo Ramothwala
Director: Positive Convention Network / July 2012

The age-old saying does not go: "It's *men*'s world". Instead, the adage asserts: "It's *a man*'s world", as though there exists only one kind of man. While it is true that men own the bulk of the world's property and occupy the majority of its leadership positions, taking a different view of this cliché makes for valuable insight into the narrow confines in which masculinity is defined.[1]

The "man" whose world it is, is an archetype – a rigidly defined image of someone who demands dominance and exudes machismo and sexual prowess.[2] This has elicited many arguments from scholars and advocates of gender equality that men are as boxed in by conventional expectations of gender roles as women.[3] *(Un)covering Men* is born from an attempt to break away from this clichéd notion to see whether it is possible to create journalism that covers different men, differently.[4]

Between 2009 and 2011, journalism fellows of the HIV & AIDS Media Project undertook in-depth research in order to write about men, masculinity and HIV in a new way. The result is this compendium of articles that showcases a diversity of men – each facing a different context and dealing with sexual health and relationships differently. Structured around four central themes, the sections in this book bring men's varied roles in the HIV epidemic to the fore – men as lovers, men as partners and fathers, men who have sex with men, and men's relationship to traditional and medical male circumcision.

1   See, for instance, UNWOMEN (2011:108).

2   Connell's (2001) seminal work on masculinities introduced the concept of one pervasive, hegemonic masculinity that dominates other subordinated or marginalised masculinities.

3   Mane and Aggleton (2001).

4   Jobson and Gibbs (2011), in their assessment of narratives of masculinity in the *Daily Sun*, found that much of the media coverage of men can be seen as an attempt to reconcile lived experiences of masculinity with dominant and traditional ideas around manhood.

By recounting different experiences, the journalism throws bare how men's ongoing struggle to negotiate expectations of what it means to be "a man" often elicits behaviour that is deeply unhealthy. In the South African context, this struggle is made even harder by a context that has biased men towards chauvinism, misogyny and homophobia.[5]

Thus for Sizwe, in Willemien Brümmer's series on lovers, maintaining multiple partnerships is a matter of "filling his father's shoes", who had four wives and multiple lovers on the side; while Hendrik, in Pieter van Zyl's *Brokeback Marriage*, chooses to suppress his attraction to men as he buckles under the pressure to maintain the façade of a "family man". In Mthetho Tshemese's journalism, the traditional circumcision attendants' choice of breakfast is informed mainly by concerns around what will make them "erect and ready", while the initiates themselves boast about their newly circumcised penises and banter about taking their "Mercedes" for a test drive. As they seek to reaffirm that they are "real men", or struggle to come to terms with their own alternative masculinity, all these men are exposed to high HIV risk.

In addition to encouraging sexual risk-taking, men's subscription to conventional masculine ideals also makes them reluctant to access health care – something they tend to consider as "sissy stuff".[6] It is this notion that eventually costs Thokozile's father his life in Thabisile Dlamini's "Hope Died with Him".[7] The research also tells us that South African men prefer to leave safe sex discussions and concerns

---

5   Morrell (2001:33).

6   Courtenay (2000).

7   An example of this attitude manifesting in its most extreme form is the view expressed by Namibian men in a focus group that being HIV positive, or even dying of AIDS-related illnesses, is the ultimate declaration of virility and thus manliness (Brown, Sorrell and Raffaelli, 2005).

to their female partners; are reluctant to test for HIV; are less likely than women to access antiretroviral treatment (ART); and present to clinics much later into their illness.[8]

Towards healthy media images of men

Truly (Un)covering Men is no easy task. The fellows were afforded the luxury of time and support that allowed them to produce these nuanced accounts of men that could take into consideration how masculine ideals impact men's health and sexual risk-taking behaviour.

This is a far cry from the environment in which most journalists are required to function. Despite immense deadline pressure and the strain placed on them by limited resources, journalists often churn out two to four stories a day. As the finer details are forced to fall by the wayside, portrayals of men (and women) often tend towards the stereotypical. Position this within the already technically and ethically dense field of HIV, and accurate and nuanced reporting becomes a tall order for any journalist.

These challenges underlie the HIV & AIDS Media Project's mission – providing journalists with the resources and skills necessary to create accurate and in-depth media coverage, particularly as it relates to HIV. The project was founded in 2003 by Anton Harber and Helen Struthers and is a joint initiative between the Journalism Programme at the University of the Witwatersrand and the Anova Health Institute. Natalie Ridgard coordinated the project from its inception to 2008, and again from 2009. In 2010 Melissa Meyer took over leadership of the project.

---

8   See Johnson (2012); Cornell, McIntyre and Myer (2011); Mindry, Maman, Chirowodza, Muravha, Van Rooyen and Coates (2011) and Nattrass (2008).

Integral to this initiative was the annual hosting of fellowships for journalists seeking to hone their skills. A changing media environment and shifts in funding objectives led to the culmination of the fellowships in 2011, but the project continues to support local media in innovative and responsive ways. This includes hosting an online resource for media professionals called journAIDS and an open hotline offering individualised support to journalists seeking specialist input. The project also promotes closer interaction between the media and medical and research professionals through discussion forums and workshops.

Part of the project's work includes daily monitoring and critical analysis of HIV media coverage to gauge the news environment and to ensure the project's support to journalists remains appropriate. This work includes ongoing consideration of how men are being covered in the context of HIV.

Positioning the fellows' journalism within this broader media context goes a long way in showing how resource availability can impact the quality of journalism and, more specifically, how it informs the manner in which men are being written about. To this end, each of the four sections in this book includes an overview of current media coverage of men relating to the particular topic.

Collectively, the components in this book make a convincing case for finding new and different ways to cover men's health issues in the media. This suggests breaking away from stereotypes and, instead, treating men as complex individuals whose behaviour is informed not only by their own notions of what it means to be a man but also by their communities, their families, their culture and, at times, also the media.

Analysis of media coverage: A brief outline of the methodology

For the media analysis contained in each section, a key word search was conducted on the HIV & AIDS Media Project's database, which contains all major print news media articles that mention HIV. The period of interest for the analysis was one year, beginning March 2011 and ending February 2012. Eleven publications were selected for the discussion, comprising the major news titles circulating in Gauteng (both dailies and weeklies), and reaching a collective readership of 16 469 000.

Name of publication	Readership
Daily Sun	5 220 000
Sunday Times	3 659 000
Sunday Sun	2 416 000
The Sowetan	1 618 000
City Press	1 604 000
The Star	576 000
Mail & Guardian	383 000
Citizen	379 000
The Times	313 000
Saturday Star	234 000
Sunday Independent	67 000
The New Age	No statistics available

Source: SAARF, 2011.

The primary data set was drawn up by cross-referencing the HIV & AIDS Media Project's database with a set of key words determined by the four themes of this book. As the HIV & AIDS Media Project's database contains only articles that make mention of HIV or AIDS, this data set was limited to articles in which HIV or AIDS were already a theme. As a result, certain data subsets were stronger than others.

Particularly, articles dealing with men who have sex with men in the context of HIV were fairly common, while articles that mentioned both fatherhood and HIV were extremely rare. This necessitated the consideration of articles mentioning HIV where men ought to have been included and articles about men where HIV should have been mentioned. The collection of this secondary data set was mostly done via the University of the Free State's media library, available from www.sabinet.co.za. Where needed, this was supplemented with a search of certain publications' online archives. Where applicable, these processes are outlined in further detail in each of the discussions.

A qualitative content analysis was subsequently conducted on the collected articles, and the information was arranged into thematic networks.[9] This allowed for the easy identification of themes and trends in the coverage. The discussions in the various sections are thus a discussion of the major trends that emerged from the news coverage.

9   Attride-Stirling (2001).

References /

Attride-Stirling, J. (2001) "Thematic networks: An analytic tool for qualitative research." *Qualitative Research*, 1(385).

Brown, J; Sorrell, J; and Raffaelli, M. (2005) "An exploratory study of constructions of masculinity, sexuality and HIV/AIDS in Namibia, Southern Africa." *Culture, Health & Sexuality*, 7(6).

Campbell, C and Gibbs, A. (2008) "Representations of HIV/AIDS management in South African newspapers." *African Journal of AIDS Research*, 7(2).

Connell, RW. (2001) "The Social Organization of Masculinity." In Whitehead, SM and Barrett, FJ (eds.). *The Masculinities Reader*. Cambridge: Polity Press.

Cornell, M; McIntyre, J; and Myer, L. (2011) "Men and antiretroviral therapy in Africa: Our blind spot." *Topical Medicine and International Health*, 16(7).

Courtenay, WH. (2000) "Engendering health: A social constructionist examination of men's health beliefs and behaviours." *Psychology of Men and Masculinity*, 1(10).

Gibbs, A and Jobson, G. (2011) "Narratives of masculinity in the *Daily Sun*: Implications for HIV risk and prevention." *South African Journal of Psychology*, 41(2).

Johnson, LF. (2012) "Access to Antiretroviral Treatment in South Africa, 2004–2011." *Southern African Journal of HIV Medicine*, 13(1).

Mane, P and Aggleton, P. (2001) "Gender and HIV/AIDS: What do men have to do with it?" *Current Sociology*, 49(6).

Mindry, D; Maman, S; Chirowodza, A; Muravha, T; Van Rooyen, H; and Coates, T. (2011) "Looking to the future: South African men and women negotiating HIV risk and relationship intimacy." *Culture, Health & Sexuality*, 13(5).

Morill, AC and Noland, C. (2010) "Interpersonal issues surrounding HIV counseling and testing, and the phenomenon of 'testing by proxy'." *Journal of Health Communication*, 11(2), 183–198.

Morell, R. (2001) *Changing Men in Southern Africa*. London: Zed Books.

Nattrass N. (2008) "Gender and access to antiretroviral treatment in South Africa." *Fem Econ* 14(4), 19–36.

South African Advertising Research Foundation (SAARF). (2011) "AMPS Jul '10–Jun '11: Average issue readership of newspapers and magazines." Retrieved 16 March 2012, http://www.saarf.co.za.

UNWOMEN. (2011) "2011–2012 Progress of the World's Women: In Pursuit of Justice." United Nations Entity for Gender Equality and the Empowerment of Women. Retrieved 10 May 2012, http://progress.unwomen.org.

Acknowledgements /

There are many organisations and individuals who contributed generously to the production and publication of this book and to the work of the HIV & AIDS Media Project on the whole. While we cannot thank everyone here, there are those of whom we need to make special mention.

First and foremost, we are extremely grateful to the project's primary donors, the United States Agency for International Development (USAID) and Johns Hopkins Health and Education in South Africa (JHHESA), through the President's Emergency Plan for AIDS Relief (PEPFAR). A big thank you goes specifically to JHHESA's former director Patrick Coleman, as well as Richard Delate who has taken over in his stead.

Our partnership with the Wits Journalism Programme has placed us in the fortunate position to work with some of the country's leading media experts. Specifically, the project's co-founder and co-director, Anton Harber, has had a pivotal role to play in providing strategic direction and support throughout the years. Joanne Richards worked intensively with the three 2009 fellows, guiding them towards the production of sophisticated and moving pieces of narrative journalism.

We are extremely grateful to all staff at the Anova Health Institute who have provided invaluable administrative and human resources support to the project since we moved there in 2009. Specific thanks are due to Anova's executive director, James McIntyre, and Glenn de Swardt from Anova's Health4Men initiative who was an important contact point for Pieter van Zyl.

Natalie Ridgard, who coordinated the project from 2004 to 2007 and again from 2009 to 2010, was pivotal in the production of the 2009 fellows' journalism research, guiding them through the research and writing process.

Ruth Becker has delivered sage advice and provided invaluable feedback during the drafting of the introductory sections. Thank you.

Kim Johnson, the project's writer, made a noteworthy contribution to the research and writing of some the introductory chapters, specifically the sections on Lovers and Fathers & Partners.

A big thank you also goes to Najma Desai, the project's administrative assistant, who methodically collected and compiled HIV-related media coverage for the analysis.

The medical officers at Cecilia Makiwane Hospital in Mdantsane provided Mthetho Tshemese with valuable assistance while he was researching traditional male circumcision.

The staff at Jacana Media, particularly Russell Clarke, have supported our initiative with enthusiasm and were key in realising our vision to produce this book. Thank you.

We are also grateful to Nardus Engelbrecht and Lebohang Mashiloane, whose photography brought life to some of the masculinities showcased here.

Finally, we must thank the fellows who approached their research with such passion and without whom *(Un)covering Men* would not have been possible.

Melissa Meyer & Helen Struthers

Lovers

"I wanted to know: 'Why don't you just leave me, rather than abuse me like this?' He said: 'I don't abuse you. My forefathers had many women.' That hurt, but I got used to it."

"I asked her: 'How could you go for the test without asking me?' I pushed her away, got in the taxi and left her. She kept phoning me, but I switched off my phone and got a new sim card. If she has the virus, it means she slept around."

Lovers / Introduction

Willemien Brümmer rewrites the script on men in the journalism featured in this chapter. For her HIV & AIDS Media Project fellowship in 2010, Brümmer returned to the sea of single HIV-positive moms in clinics and hospitals who had piqued her interest during a previous assignment. With the scope and resources the fellowship afforded her, Brümmer set out to investigate why men leave "when HIV comes to stay". What she discovered was an exceedingly complex issue, exacerbated by denial, sexual infidelity, violence and the asphyxiating poverty that creeps through the cracks of already fragile relationships.

True to the realities she uncovered, Brümmer's series features men who go *and* men who stay. With a set of four heartrending and sometimes hopeful vignettes, she shares the experiences of a number of lovers. But her stories do not only probe the "what" – by peeling back the personal narratives, the journalism throws bare the social issues that underpin these men's actions, offering a rare moment of insight into the intricacies that are at play in relationships when men attempt to live up to certain masculine ideals.

This is achieved skilfully by telling Sizwe's story in "Hush, brother, there goes a *real* man". Blending Sizwe's experiences with research and expert commentary, Brümmer sketches a detailed account of how masculine ideals around sexual virility, strength and dominance feed into risky sexual behaviours and foster an overall unwillingness to seek medical care.[1] For Sizwe, and many other young men, sexual prowess or being "a stud" is considered a key trait of being a real man.[2] In Sizwe's own words: "Men should always have two or three women". When Brümmer asks Sizwe about safe sex, it becomes clear

1   Courtenay (2000).

2   Wood and Jewkes (2001).

how this adherence to dominant masculine ideals is endangering his health: "Real men don't use condoms," he responds.

The stranglehold of these narrowly defined ideas around what makes a man, a man, not only takes its toll on men's use of HIV-prevention methods but also negatively affects their readiness to access HIV treatment.[3,4] Thus Sizwe remains adamant that HIV does not exist and he, like many other men, repeatedly refuses to go for an HIV test.[5] Trapped by his own notion that a real man must at all times have the upper hand, he refuses to connect the dots between his girlfriend's HIV diagnosis and his own status. Instead, he lashes out, scorning her for infidelity and disobedience, despite his own inability to remain faithful.

But the story of Sizwe also investigates the potential for men to change by offering a protagonist in the form of Mbulelo Zuba, who is living openly with HIV. Mbulelo is encouraging his friend Sizwe to face up to the reality of HIV and get tested. In the end, it is Mbulelo who is ultimately framed as the "real" man, one who faces up to his choices and takes care of his sexual health.

Following Sizwe's story is that of Vusumzi. Like Sizwe, Vusumzi is *indoda ebalekileyo*, the man who ran away, and like Sizwe, Vusumzi also grew up during a period in South Africa's history made infamous for AIDS denialism among the top echelons of government.[6] Although both men have a history of multiple and concurrent partnerships, Vusumzi's trail of women and children is so exten-

3   Galdas, Cheater and Marshall (2005).

4   Kigozi, Dobkin, Martin, Geng, Muyindike, Emenyonu, Bangsberg and Hahn (2009).

5   According to a recent study conducted in Soweto by Venkatesh, Madiba, De Bruyn, Lurie, Coates and Gray (2011), 68.4 per cent of women reported that they had tested for HIV. In comparison, only 28.9 per cent of men said that they had had an HIV test sometime in the past.

6   See Fourie and Meyer (2010).

sive that a chronological account of his many relationships and the four children he has with four different women forms the backbone of his story.

This timeline reveals overlapping relationships and, in so doing, illustrates the full scale of the HIV risk inherent in multiple and concurrent partnerships like these. But Vusumzi's various partners were as unaware of this overlap as they were of his HIV status. Though Vusumzi first learned he was HIV positive in his final year at school, it would take decades, numerous partnerships and four children later before his journey became one of acceptance, treatment and disclosure.

Despite the many lies that held Vusumzi's relationships together, he is not devoid of conscience. Through detailed narrative accounts, Brümmer reveals a man tormented by guilt, to whom running away often seemed the only option. "Every time I saw her she was in pain. I couldn't handle it," is his justification for leaving Sindiswa after she discovered that she had contracted HIV (most likely from him) and was pregnant with his child.

By granting airtime to the man who left, Brümmer does something rarely achieved in coverage of men – she elicits empathy through insight. Through sharing Vusumzi's side of the story, she takes the stereotypical absconding lover and renders him not a villain, but rather another causality claimed when HIV enters relationships.

In keeping with Brümmer's judicious and comprehensive approach, one of the stories of men who leave is told from a woman's perspective. In "Not a dog's sickness", we meet Sarie Sineli, who has been abandoned by her husband because, according to him, she "brought HIV into the house". Sarie's story has all the hallmarks of the others but is important as a counterpoint to the men's narratives.

Sarie's struggle to single-handedly fend for her family brings the desperation of poverty to the fore, which exists as a quiet undercurrent in the other narratives as well. Though Sarie's continuing love for, and loyalty to, her husband are heartbreaking, her battle with substance abuse and depression remind the reader that when lovers part, clear lines between victims and perpetrators are not easily drawn.

The last and most redemptive story in Brümmer's collection is that of Lester: an HIV-negative man standing by his desperately ill HIV-positive wife, Katy, and their two children, who both are positive. Lester's willingness to assume the caregiver role, which men usually shy away from, is proof that men can and do adopt emancipatory forms of masculinity.[7] Though, as our analysis will show, these images of men as caregivers are exceptionally rare.

Like Sarie, it is now Lester who battles to be the breadwinner and the caregiver, offering a view of how HIV and poverty intersect in South Africa.[8] Through Lester's animated character, Brümmer is able to convey his resilience and patience with his ailing wife and sickly children. While Lester says he is now "mommy and daddy" to the children, he does not consider his role as caregiver emasculating. Much of this is probably informed by the example set by Lester's father, who himself took on a lot of the housework after Lester's mother had a stroke. Unlike the other men in Brümmer's stories, Lester's father was also a man who stayed after illness and hardship descended.

The true tragedy of Lester's story, however, is one of a great love lost. While Lester's devotion to his wife lives on through his caregiving, very little remains of the boisterous woman he once adored. But Lester has chosen to "man up" to his fate and, in the bravest declaration of manliness made in Brümmer's work, he asserts: "This is the cross I have to bear – and it's a cast-iron cross, you know".

7   Morrell (2001).

8   Whiteside (2002).

Current coverage: Hard-and-fast media images of men as lovers

In the year-long period spanned by our analysis, media coverage of men as lovers in the context of HIV was considerably less nuanced and detailed than the journalism showcased here. As a result, news reports were highly likely to pigeonhole men as Lotharios and vectors of disease in the context of HIV. On the other hand, coverage of women and HIV does not appear to ameliorate the situation either, often enforcing this man-woman, vector-victim dichotomy.[9]

A total of 47 articles was sourced through searches of the HIV & AIDS Media Project's database, using keywords relating to the topics men, sex, love, relationships and men's sexual health.[10,11] Following a close reading, the articles in this sample were divided into five organising themes: multiple concurrent partnerships (MCP); intergenerational sex or "sugar daddies"; alleged intentional or reckless transmission of HIV; Zulu and Swati reed dances; and HIV testing.

He loves to get around: Men in multiple and concurrent partnerships, sugar daddies and "dogs"

In our analysis, where the media covered men as lovers in the context of HIV, there was a marked tendency to appropriate blame. Four of

---

9   See, for example, Ramjee's "Women are the vulnerable HIV link" (*Mail & Guardian*, December 2011). The headline, along with the picture of a visibly ill woman being spoon-fed, perpetuates the disempowering notion that women are hapless victims when it comes to HIV.

10   Given the limitations of the HIV & AIDS Media Project's database, which only includes HIV-related coverage, the University of the Free State's database was used to supplement searches where necessary.

11   The high number of reed-dance articles turned up through our searches necessitated further investigation and the widening of search parameters to include these articles.

the five organising themes engaged with some form of vector-victim dichotomy and, of those, three clearly blamed men. Most prominent among these was the coverage of men in MCP. Notably, the bulk of this category was made up of coverage on local sports minister Fikile Mbalula's reportedly unprotected trysts with a model in October 2011, which accounted for 9 of 12 reports. Mbalula's standing as a high-profile political figure who, ironically, supported the government's ABC (abstain, be faithful, condomise) campaign, most likely contributed to the news value of this story.

The rest of the MCP coverage consisted of an equal mix of personal true-life accounts and news reports. Both of the personal narratives in the sample emphasised risky sexual behaviour in the context of manliness, but while one took a cautionary stance, the other seemed to promote MCP as a prized quality among "real" men. In the first article, *Bona* magazine profiles Khumo Khumo as a "zero convert" who has not contracted HIV despite having multiple HIV-positive partners. The aptly titled "Dicing with death" is a laundry list of unprotected sexual encounters, revealing complex webs of sexual activity.[12] The article ends on a cautionary note, with Khumo's acknowledgement of the dangers in which he has put himself and his partners. On the other side of the coin is a *Daily Sun* article on local personality Sithembele Maswana.[13] In awe-inspired tones, Maswana is made out to be a hyper-masculine hunter with a voracious sexual appetite and the ability to have "long, hard sessions" with an infinite number of sexual partners.

The remaining two articles in the MCP category were news reports both featuring health minister Aaron Motsoaledi's rebuking of "immoral men" and husbands, blaming them for the high rate of

12   "Dicing with death", *Bona* (March 2012).

13   Sizani, M. "Super 4–5!", *Daily Sun* (September 2011).

HIV among older women.[14,15] Interestingly, these two articles did not draw from one event or one statement but were published months apart in June 2011 and November 2011.

The second-most common theme to frame men as lovers comprised coverage of men engaging in intergenerational sex. All of the reports in this category examined the dangers of these relationships, although some focused on teen pregnancy to the detriment of the HIV issue. The majority of these directly and indirectly tackled the topic of "sugar daddies" – older men who have sex with younger women. One article touched on intergenerational sex in the context of *ukuthwala*, the practice of abducting young girls and coercing them into marrying older men.[16]

Coverage of the sugar daddy issue was for the most part simplistic, making no attempt to probe the conditions and causes that give rise to sugar daddy relationships.[17,18] The stories also tended to lay the blame for HIV and teen pregnancy entirely at the feet of men. Most articles conveyed the message that the young women involved were usually "coerced" into having relationships with older men.

But it was not all bad news. One article in *The New Age* took a more considered approach.[19] Speaking to young girls, the report revealed that women often actively seek out sugar daddy relationships for many reasons, not limited to material gain. Another article in *The Citizen* included intergenerational sex in a story on getting

14   Mabuza, K. "Immoral men in the HIV spotlight", *Sowetan* (June 2011).

15   McLea, H. "Husbands a 'big problem'", *The Times* (November 2011).

16   Odendal, L. "Forcing the issue", *Mail & Guardian* (April 2011).

17   Khambule, L and Dlungwana, M. "There's nothing sweet about sugar daddies!", *Daily Sun* (January 2012).

18   Singh, A. "Curse of the sugar daddies", *Daily Sun* (January 2012).

19   Dube, D. "Anti-sugar daddy drive launched", *The New Age* (January 2012).

basic feminine toiletries to underprivileged young girls, touching on the socio-economic context that informs these behaviours.[20] But while theses reports provide some insight into the conditions of women and girls, they continue to frame men in a very one-dimensional manner.

In the third major theme, reed dances, coverage again exhibited an element of blame – in this case, that men alone were at fault for a rise in sex before marriage among maidens. However, rather than being castigated outright, men were more subtly referred in negative terms like "hormone driven".[21] Stronger criticism was voiced by women and cultural groups quoted as saying men who "robbed" the women of their virginity were "dogs" and that the virgin maidens needed to be protected.[22,23] In all these articles, the voices of men were glaringly absent. In so doing, not only did the articles fail to hold men accountable, they also failed in getting to the crux of the matter through balanced reporting.

The fourth theme in our analysis, of alleged intentional or reckless transmission of HIV, was the only one where the roles of victim and vector could be reversed and women were at times "blamed" for HIV transmission. Three of the five articles in this category covered the same case. These articles featured the vignette of a doctor whose wife had allegedly knowingly infected him with HIV.[24,25,26] Another

20 Health reporter. "Girls receive feminine care packages", *The Citizen* (September 2011).

21 Mooki, O. "When virginity and virtue go hand in hand", *The Star* (November 2011).

22 Masuku, S. "Maidens appeal to king of Zulus", *Sowetan* (June 2011).

23 Mooki, O. "When virginity and virtue go hand in hand", *The Star* (November 2011)

24 Chauke, A. "She infected me, says doc", *The Times* (September 2011).

25 Moselakgomo, A. "My wife infected me with HIV, says doctor", *Sowetan* (September 2011).

26 Makgalemele, T. "Lovesick", *Drum* (October 2011).

report told the story of a young woman who infected men as revenge for her contracting the virus through rape. The final piece in the category was the story of a group of women who had all been infected by a "deadly seducer".[27]

Men's health and HIV

Only one category in our analysis could be considered to have broken away from the vector-victim trend. Unlike the four preceding themes, this fifth category did not contribute to the "men-as-vectors" argument but rather took a more positive approach, reporting on men's poor health-seeking behaviour in connection with HIV testing.[28,29]

Regrettably, of the five reports in this category that focused on men's lack of interest in HIV testing, most articles simply regurgitated facts drawn from government reports and documents. This meant that they provided little added insight into why men are less likely than women to seek help. Only one article took a more insightful stance, with the male writer talking about his own personal struggles with HIV testing in an attempt to shed light on why it is that men generally avoid it.[30]

Also included in this category were articles reporting on the death of Bafana Bafana soccer star Thabang Lebese, who died from

27   Waterworth, T. "Women tell of 'deadly seducer'", www.iol.co.za (January 2012).

28   Mashaba, S. "SA men urged to get tested for HIV", *Sowetan* (December 2011).

29   Tlhakudi, M. "Men need to test for HIV", *Sowetan* (August 2011).

30   Mukundu, R. "Men need to stop being scared of testing", *The New Age* (December 2011).

an AIDS-related illness.[31,32,33] Although Lebese's death from a chronic but manageable condition provided the media with the opportunity to address men's poor health-seeking behaviour, the issue was never broached.

Given the clamour around women's disproportionate HIV burden, men's roles as lovers of women are frequently overlooked in HIV programmes. Perhaps spurred on by this inequality, media images tend to be reductive, frequently positioning women as hapless victims and men as perpetrators. The journalism showcased in this section is evidence that it is possible to circumvent this vector-victim binary by writing about both men and women as stakeholders in relationships and providing insight and context.

Though what the journalism showcased here also points to is that many men still cling desperately to dominant masculine ideals that put both their and their partners' health at stake. This suggests that much work lies ahead in changing men's ideas around how "real" men behave in relationships and, particularly, in the context of HIV.

31   Molefe, M. "Lebese 'died of Aids'", *The Times* (March 2012).

32   Seale, L. "Family reveals hidden truth", *The Star* (March 2012).

33   Molefe, M. "Lebese had AIDS", *Sowetan* (March 2012).

References /

Courtenay, W. (2000) "Constructions of masculinity and their influence on men's well-being: A theory of gender and health." *Social Science & Medicine*, 50, 1385–1401.

Fourie, P and Meyer, M. (2010) *The Politics of AIDS Denialism: South Africa's failure to respond*. London: Ashgate.

Galdas, P; Cheater, F; and Marshall, P. (2005) "Men and health help-seeking behaviour: Literature review." *Journal of Advanced Nursing*, 49(6), 616–623.

Jobson, G and Gibbs, A. (2011) "Narratives of masculinity in the *Daily Sun*: Implications for HIV risk and prevention." *South African Journal of Psychology*, 41 (2), 173–186.

Kigozi, I; Dobkin, L; Martin, J; Geng, E; Muyindike, W; Emenyonu, N; Bangsberg, D; and Hahn, J. (2009) "Late disease stage at presentation to an HIV clinic in the era of free antiretroviral therapy in sub-Saharan Africa." *Journal of Acquired Immune Deficiency Syndrome*, 52(2), 280.

MacPhail, C and Campbell, C. (2001) "'I think condoms are good but, aai, I hate those things': Condom use among adolescents and young people in a southern African township." *Social Science & Medicine*, 52(11), 1613–1627.

Morrell, R. (2001) *Changing Men in Southern Africa*. Pietermaritzburg: University of Natal Press.

Venkatesh, K; Madiba, P; De Bruyn, G; Lurie, M; Coates, T; and Gray, G. (2011) "Who Gets tested for HIV in a South African urban township? Implications for test and treat and gender-based prevention interventions." *Journal of Acquired Immune Deficiency Syndrome*, 56(2).

Whiteside, A. (2002) "Poverty and HIV/AIDS in Africa." *Third World Quarterly*, 23(2), 313–332.

Wood, K and Jewkes, R. (2001) "'Dangerous' love: Reflections on violence among Xhosa township youth." In Morrell, R (ed.) *Changing men in Southern Africa*. Pietermaritzburg: University of Natal Press and London: Zed Press.

Lovers / Journalism

Where have all the fathers gone?

Willemien Brümmer

In Xhosa the women simply say *le ndoda ibalekile* – this man, he ran away.

In a time of HIV and AIDS, this story has virtually become a template – a cultural narrative etched into countless women's minds: She tests positive for HIV; her husband blames her for "bringing AIDS into the house"; he packs up and leaves.

In the paediatric AIDS Unit at Groote Schuur Hospital in Observatory, where I completed a research project in 2005, 9 out of 10 HIV-positive mothers I interviewed were single. When I returned to visit the unit again in 2010, the women told the same story: one of HIV and abandonment.

The up side? Some men eventually come back.

One woman, Nombeko (not her real name), was so angry when she found the father of her disabled son (at that time two years old) in bed with another woman that she shouted, "We're all HIV positive! Now you'll give it to her!"

"It's you and your baby, I'm not positive," he countered. "Stay with your AIDS baby," he said and left.

When the toddler turned four, his father fell ill and started bringing Nombeko money. As time passed, he asked sheepishly: "Nombeko, please can I go with you to Groote Schuur Hospital? I also want to see the doctor."

Nombeko frowns, rolls her eyes. "He still insisted that he was negative, but when he later moved in with us, he changed his story. He said 'sorry.'"

Pumla Tyulu, a counsellor at the paediatric AIDS unit, estimates that up to 80 per cent of the mothers who bring their children here are single.

"The mothers often say that when they disclosed their status, their husband or boyfriend ran away and started an affair or went and found a new girlfriend," says Tyulu. "After a while the mother would find a new partner, but she usually struggles to disclose that she is HIV positive, because she is afraid he too will leave. It's a vicious cycle. The women always say our children grow up without a father because of HIV and AIDS."

The Sinomlando Centre for Oral History and Memory Work inverviewed 33 families in KwaZulu-Natal who were affected by the virus. Only 27 per cent of the fathers in these families had regular contact with their children. About 34 per cent of them provided some sort of material support. The rest? They were simply never mentioned.

But why *do* the fathers leave?

In April 2010 I started investigating how men react when their life partner or the mother of their children admits that she is HIV positive. I interviewed more than 20 men and women living with HIV, as well as experts, counsellors and activists. I found that love obeys no rules, and that the truth is a murky zone, an in-between land where neither men nor women reign supreme.

I talked to HIV-negative men who stay with women and children living with the virus despite society's taboos, and to men who believe this illness "only exists in white people's minds".

Often the relationship had been shaky before the man left. HIV was simply the penultimate chapter in a relationship characterised by poverty and violence.

Some names have been changed.

"Not a dog's sickness"

Willemien Brümmer

When Sarie Sineli found out she had the virus, her husband "just vanished" and changed his phone number. Today she asks the Lord to make him come back. "He wasn't good to me, but I had food," she explains. "He packed his clothes and he left."

The winter rain flings surges of freezing-cold sleet at Mama Mable Solani's bedroom windows. Sarie (not her real name) pulls her threadbare beige jersey tightly around her shoulders. Her body is thin and wasted like that of a feral kitten. One of countless women summoned by Mama Solani to sit in the "confessional chair" in her bedroom, hers was the umpteenth tale of HIV and rejection.

Just like the others, Sarie (45) attends the weekly HIV support group that is part of Mama Solani's Helping Hands Project, run from her double-storey house in KTC, a township close to Nyanga, Cape Town. But Sarie doesn't only come to be counselled. She knocks on Mable's front door so that she and her children (14 and 18) can eat.

Earlier today, a 58-year-old mother of three, her face painted white, wearing a blue chintz skirt, walked into the bedroom. It's the last space in Mama Solani's house not infested with screaming children, volunteers or singing women. The mother unknotted her headscarf to reveal the shiny scars on her face. Her ankle bore the signs of surgery.

"I had to go to the Conradie Hospital in Pinelands," she explained, her tone unwavering. She did not seem sorry for herself. Her dark eyes had found peace. "There were gashes on my head and he broke my ankle."

Like many of her "sisters" at Mama Solani's, she spoke of the other women in her husband's life. After 20 years of marriage she went for an HIV test. Her worst fears were confirmed.

The woman bit her lip. "He assaulted me, because he blamed me and said that I had brought the virus into our house. He did not want to get tested. He packed up and moved in with another girlfriend."

Those brown eyes remained stoic: "I never see him; I don't know where he is. I think he is probably still alive – no one has told me that he has died."

Her lips curve upwards. "I have nothing against him; I let him go."

This mother of three has been on her own for 14 years now. She never again let a man into her life, because she doesn't want to "become reinfected," she says.

For Sarie everything is still raw and new.

Sitting on the same confessional chair as her predecessor, she tells how her life has changed since she was diagnosed with HIV last year. Unlike most of the other women, she doesn't need an interpreter. Born in Prieska, she speaks a textured Northern Cape Afrikaans.

"I was an outpatient at GF Jooste Hospital [in Manenberg] for my high blood [pressure], and they tested me for HIV," she says. The results did not shock her. "I knew this illness wasn't a dog's sickness, it's anyone's sickness. I came home and saw my sister, and I thought of how pretty she was. She's also HIV positive. She's fat – I thought I'll just do what she's doing."

But when Sarie told her husband, Gerald (not his real name), to whom she'd been married for 22 years, the news obliterated the last certainties in an uncertain marriage.

She looks outside at the carefree toddlers running around on wobbly legs in Mama Solani's crèche. "I told my husband I was positive and then he yelled *I* brought this illness. He said he didn't have AIDS, *I* did. He just vanished; he didn't even say where he was going."

She soon learned that he had moved in with another woman.

Sarie, already unemployed at the time, threatened to put the police on him. "I wanted him to at least pay maintenance for the kids." Yet all he had left behind was the simple one-bedroomed house about a block from Mama Solani's where Sarie and her two children, and her sister and her baby, still live.

She casts her gaze downward. "I never saw him again. I don't know where he is. He changed his phone number. Not even his children hear from him."

In the months that followed, I pieced together the rest of Sarie's story. It started 45 years ago in Prieska where she grew up as "a wild child that didn't have a dad". Her Afrikaans-speaking mother worked for white people in Sea Point and sent money home so that Sarie's grandmother could look after her and her four brothers and sisters. Sarie's Tswana-speaking father had no contact with his children.

"My grandma hit us and hurt us," Sarie remembers. It's the end of August in Mama Solani's bedroom. Outside it is a crisp and joyous Friday. Women are praying, dancing and singing, hands lifted high. Mama Solani has just handed them their monthly food parcels.

Sarie left school in Standard Five and moved to Cape Town at the age of 20. The romance with Gerald began when she needed 50 cents to travel from the squatter camp in KTC to her work in Sea Point.

"I asked my neighbour for the money and he asked Gerald. Gerald put the money in his mouth and told me I had to kiss him to get the 50 cents." She smiles. "When I got home that night he said: 'I love you.' I fancied him from the start."

Silence. "Now I'm trying to forget."

About three months after they'd met, Gerald took Sarie to his family in the Eastern Cape for a traditional wedding.

"When I got there, I couldn't speak Xhosa very well, and my mother-in-law called me a *Boesmanmeid*." A cow and a goat were slaughtered and Sarie learned to carry water on her head and how to fetch wood to make a fire.

Back home in KTC the problems began. She lifts her skirt to show me a shiny mark on her leg. "Once when he was drunk he took one of the bedposts and hit my right leg. I had to go to hospital. My sister said: 'This man will kill you one day,' but I said: 'I love him.'"

She sighs, her head held high. "The hitting was better than the words. He makes you his floor rag."

It wasn't long before he started leaving her alone at night to go to sleep with other women. If she dared to question him, he hit her.

"I wanted to know: 'Why don't you just leave me, rather than abuse me like this?' He said: 'I don't abuse you. My forefathers had many women.' That hurt, but I got used to it."

She reflects for a moment. "I was afraid of HIV. If a man is doing his rounds like that, how can I not also have the thing? When we had sex, he never wanted condoms. He wanted to go with the flesh."

Two years ago one of the women in his life died due to AIDS-related causes. "I heard it from other people, he didn't tell me himself," Sarie remembers. "I told him we must go for the test together, but he refused. He said *I* was the sick one – that I was sleeping around." She makes a clicking noise with her tongue. "He sees me every morning when I open the door of our house to him – I iron his clothes and I make his food. I don't sleep around and I look after the children."

Since her own diagnosis, she has met some of his other girlfriends at the clinic. "They're also ill, I saw them getting the pills. Fortunately, mine isn't that bad yet. Just my heart and the high blood pressure."

She tells me that one day her husband's brother came to her house. He came to ask: "Why did Gerald run away?" she says. "His brother said Gerald was with his family in the Transkei."

She shrugs. "I said to his brother: 'Go ask Gerald why he left'."

She turns to me. "I don't think he's been tested. If you go for a test, you have to tell your family."

It is October when I stop by Mama Solani again. This time there are no women singing and praying by her front door. There is no smell of *vetkoek* in the air. "Mama Solani says there is no food," says a bewildered Sarie. She's unsteady and smells of alcohol.

"For two days now there's been no cooking here – yesterday and today," she stutters. "I'm looking after my sister's child who is a year and six months old, because my sister is with her boyfriend. Now I have to feed this child too, that's why I'm going around asking people for food. This morning I asked another woman for mealie meal, but now there's nothing in the house."

The guilt is stencilled all over her face. "My own children go to school hungry. My son said to me: 'Mama, don't worry, I'll get food at school.' The eldest is working at Steers after school."

She looks away. "I know the drinking costs money, but it was at another woman's house. She invited me for the *umqomboti* and brandy. This woman made beer for the forefathers who are dead."

Yes, she nods, sometimes she looks for work. "After my husband left I sometimes went to Cape Town for casual jobs, but now I no longer have money for the taxi." Her eyes fill up. "If he was here, I wouldn't be struggling so hard. He wasn't good to me, but I had food. And he loved his kids."

Did her husband's brother come again? She nods hesitantly. "His brother says he thinks he will come back and I must forgive him. He must be sick. I don't know how long he'll stay in the Transkei. But I'll just ask the Lord to let him come back. That's all."

She wipes her eyes with her worn-out sleeve. "If he comes, I'll take him back. It's no good for him to leave me and go and give it to someone else. He and I have to deal with it together."

Her voice is soft, I can hardly hear her. "I love him."

Some names have been changed. Originally published in Afrikaans as "Nie 'n hond se siek" on 6 November 2010 in By, *a supplement to* Die Burger, Volksblad *and* Beeld.

"Hush, brother, there goes a *real* man"

Willemien Brümmer

Miracles do happen – especially in a time of HIV and AIDS.
Willemien Brümmer spoke to the experts about leaving or staying
when the virus comes knocking.

"Her eyes became two glasses of water when she told me she had the virus," says Sizwe.

He looks away, folds his arms across his chest like a shield. His friend, Mbulelo Zuba, also from Gugulethu on the Cape Flats, spurs him on. Wearily Sizwe (not his real name) recounts his relationship with Cynthia from Nyanga East.

They met in January 2007 – "nice and fat like my mother and with big eyes and short hair". For two years and nine months they were lovers, even though he admits boastfully that at the same time he was involved with the mother of his child and yet another woman. He smiles. "My father had three wives in the Transkei. I have to fill his shoes."

He is taken aback by my question: "No, I don't use condoms. Real men don't use condoms."

The affair with Cynthia came to an abrupt end when she tested herself in September last year. She told Sizwe she was positive.

"I asked her: 'How could you go for the test without asking me?' I pushed her away, got in the taxi and left her." He frowns. "She kept phoning me, but I switched off my phone and got a new sim card. If she has the virus, it means she slept around."

In his broken English he explains haltingly: "Men should always have two or three women; there're too many women in the world and not enough men. Women may only have one."

How does he know she "slept around"?

"She cried and said she only had sex with me. I didn't want to talk about it any more. I was so angry I would've killed her if I had stayed. I don't want a girl who tells me about HIV. I don't believe in it."

He nods – yes, other "real black men" would also have left. "The Xhosa people don't like it if girls tell them they have HIV. We're different because of our traditions. When I became an *oluka* [a man], they taught me you had to be the head of the household. If your wife doesn't listen to you, you have to leave her."

He would rather die than have himself tested for HIV, he insists. "The sangomas are better. I don't want to do something that can hurt my life."

His friend Mbulelo, also the secretary of the support group Khululeka for HIV-positive men, probes, "Will you come to the clinic with me to see for yourself that I test positive?"

Sizwe's eyes grow murky. "I will go back to the Eastern Cape where nobody talks about AIDS," he says curtly. "You will no longer be my friend."

And then, suddenly, he drops the veneer. "I don't want to talk about things that make me sad. I loved Cynthia for her big eyes. I really loved her ..."

Mbulelo chimes in. "In our culture many people think HIV is a curse. If someone doesn't like you, they'll give you something to kill you. I try to make men aware of their illness, but most men think 'nobody should tell me about HIV. If I want to sleep with my wife without a condom, I will do it, because I paid *lobola* for her.' The men think it is their duty to make children, and HIV cannot stand in the way of that."

He casts an emphatic glance towards his friend.

"I've tried to convince him so many times that I am positive, but that I am healthy because of the antiretrovirals. He said: 'No, bra, don't try and convince me, I don't want to understand – I hear it is something that people over there in Zambia and Angola have'."

The reality is that Sizwe is a castaway, desperately clinging to the shipwrecked traditions of his forefathers. Together Mbulelo and Sizwe are the Dr Jekyll and Mr Hyde of the AIDS era: Sizwe resists change, while Mbulelo challenges the obdurate ideas about traditional masculinity in his community.

But how often do men decide to end a relationship because of HIV – or are stories like Sizwe's a stereotype blown out of proportion by the media (and women)? The answer is as complex as love itself.

The issue should be considered in a broader context: According to the census data of 1996, men are 10 times more inclined than women to leave their families. Often HIV is just the tip of the iceberg.

However, passing moral judgement on men who leave, particularly from a purely Western point of view, would be oversimplifying the matter. For many South Africans who grew up in well-off Christian households, the goals of a relationship are a white dress at the altar – "until death do us part" – and then a baby shower. But wordwide the institution of marriage is in crisis.

And although marriage has traditionally been a building block of "real masculinity" in many African cultures, poverty now acts as a bulldozer, razing "luxuries" such as everlasting fidelity to the ground.

Due to increasing unemployment, ever fewer men are able to afford *ilobolo* [a dowry], according to Philippe Denis and Radikobo Ntsimane writing in *Baba: Men and fatherhood in South Africa.* Many women have become sceptical about marriage – but in African culture children continue to be extremely valuable.

Population data recorded since the Second World War shows

that at least a third – in some cases up to 80 per cent – of children in black townships were born to unmarried mothers. Recent research shows that half of all black women have had a child by the time they turn 21 – and they are mostly unmarried. An overwhelming majority of South African children grow up in female-headed households.

Dr Nelis Grobbelaar, programme manager of an HIV partnership in the West Coast–Winelands region, estimates that up to 70 per cent of the HIV-positive pregnant women in his unit have not yet decided whether they want to get married to the future fathers of their newborns. "These women are expected to tell the man: 'I'm pregnant and, by the way, I'm HIV positive and the doctor says I have to take these pills for the rest of my life and I'm not allowed to breastfeed'."

Dr Grobbelaar sighs. "Nothing is normal. To reveal your status to someone you already feel uncertain about is very, very difficult. Many of the men feel they didn't ask the woman to fall pregnant in the first place, they only wanted to have sex with her."

These fragile relationships are further complicated by the notion that men should be the breadwinner. But when HIV becomes an uninvited guest, often it is not long before the money dries up.

Mbuyiselo Botha, fervent gender activist and senior programme manager of the Sonke Gender Justice Network, talks about the men he has worked with in the past 20 years. They repeatedly said, "When I am unemployed, I do not feel like a real man." In his rich baritone, he explains: "These men often feel it's better for them to leave, since there won't be unnecessary pressure to provide materially, or even to take the lead."

If the women hear about their status first, the men also do not want to be associated with something they consider to be "a death sentence", says Botha. "This is why men in many cases rather get tested 'via their sex partners'. They don't go to the testing station themselves, because a positive result leaves them feeling hopeless or powerless. Most men are raised with the idea that they have to be in control all the time. They think people will forever see them as a failure, someone who brought dishonour to the household."

Often, he says, men also do not want to spoil their chances of having other relationships. "He thinks if he is involved with an HIV-positive woman, he will also be identified as being HIV positive."

Researchers have confirmed this observation. Despite the high incidence of HIV, "most men pursue a 'successful' masculinity by having more than one sex partner," according to Sakhumzi Mfecane, an anthropologist at the University of the Western Cape. Add to this the lethal combination of risky sexual behaviour, violence and HIV, and the outlook for women is dark indeed.

In an essay titled "Gender and sexuality: Emerging perspectives from the heterosexual epidemic in South Africa and implications for HIV risk and prevention", researchers Rachel Jewkes and Robert Morrell write that there is convincing evidence that unequal relationships between men and women increase women's risk of becoming infected. In addition, women are biologically more susceptible to the virus. And an HIV-positive status is more common among men who have a history of violence towards their sexual partners than their more peaceful brethren.

For African women, they write, "excusing male behaviour is an integral part of dominant femininity and essential for keeping the right man. In a practical sense, that entails tolerance of violence, tolerance of his other partners, and ensuring that sex with the right man is 'the best' (i.e. no condoms)."

The women are also vulnerable because, for the most part, they get tested before men. This makes it easier for the man to blame the woman for "bringing the virus into the home". According to Mfecane, who recently completed his doctoral thesis on a group of HIV-positive men in Bushbuckridge, Mpumalanga, who use antiretrovirals, most women get tested at the prenatal clinics to prevent transmission of the virus to their unborn babies.

Of the 25 men in his study, all but one only got tested for HIV when they became seriously ill. Why? People with HIV in this area – especially those with visible physical symptoms – were often treated as outcasts, as though they were "already dead". Most other men in Bushbuckridge chose to keep their status a secret – or to die rather than have blood taken for a HIV test. They figured that "real men" handled their problems on their own, otherwise they would be weaklings. Being open about HIV is regarded a public acknowledgement that they had done something wrong and "immoral".

"I was told most men choose to keep silent and continue to have unprotected sex with their partners," says Mfecane.

Many of the men also have a deep-seated mistrust of Western medicine and white doctors. "They consider themselves guardians of their culture and are much more sensitive about it than women. The men felt that if they used white medicine, they were taking part in the destruction of their own culture and way of life."

The men in Bushbuckridge described the clinics as *indawo yabafati* – a place of women. Those who eventually did test positive mostly stayed mute until the antiretrovirals made them look healthier. "They did not want to talk during a 'weak phase'. They felt that if their partners left them while they were ill, there would be no one to care for them. When they felt stronger, they were more independent and able to get another woman."

Yet it is dangerous to think only men "disappear" when the virus comes knocking on the door. In Mfecane's study, four men were abandoned by their female sexual partners after the men disclosed their status. Ten women decided to stay and seven of the men had no stable partner. Three women chose to partially separate from their partners and moved in with family.

"Particularly the younger women tended to leave, but those in longer-term relationships with two or three children would not take such a decision lightly," he says. "They also reasoned that if they left, they would probably just meet another man who didn't want to use condoms. They realised the chances were good that they were also HIV positive."

The good news? The couples who stayed together mostly had a more meaningful relationship after a frank discussion about HIV. Many men decided to end their other relationships. Those who worked in distant places, such as Johannesburg, were forced to come home because of their illness. Surprisingly, many of these men also regained a degree of dignity and respect in the community after disclosing their status – precisely because they were brave enough to challenge dominant ideas of masculinity.

"Instead of being rejected and treated as outcasts, they earned respect and were regarded as 'good men' and 'role models' in their community," says Mfecane.

It is for this reason that Mbulelo Zuba says to his friend Sizwe again and again: "At first I also thought AIDS did not exist. But since I got tested, I can encourage other men to follow suit." He thrusts his chest out proudly. "I can talk in front of a million people about my status. When they see me in the location they will say: 'Hush, brother, there goes a *real* man'."

And miracles *do* happen – perhaps especially in a time of HIV and AIDS: When I spoke to Mbulelo about Sizwe again after some months, his voice was light and cheerful. "Sizwe and I are going to the clinic this weekend," Mbulelo said. "He decided to get tested."

Some names have been changed. Originally published in Afrikaans as "Stil, broer, daar stap 'n man verby" on 13 November 2010 in By, *a supplement in* Die Burger, Volksblad *and* Beeld.

Indoda ebalekileyo

Willemien Brümmer

*In his matric year, he was summoned to a home in Bonteheuwel.
He will never forget his girlfriend's words: "Vusumzi, I'm pregnant
and I found out that I'm HIV positive." Willemien Brümmer tells
the story of the man who ran away.*

"It was difficult, but I've forgiven myself," Vusumzi says, his hands
clutching at the edge of the table as though it were a witness stand
in a courtroom.

Weighty words for a man whose nickname could just as well
have been *indoda ebalekileyo* – the man who ran away.

With his jokes, boyish face and dimples, Vusumzi (33) is a
charming man, the kind you desperately want to believe. Yet I had
to discover the truth about him in a roundabout way. For weeks,
even months, he'd shy away from appointments. When we did meet,
our conversations felt like small islands of understanding scattered
across a dark and vast ocean. On parting he would each and every
time mutter: "secrets hurt – the talking clears my heart."

Myra and Valerie

It is June and endless sheets of rain fall down upon the Cape Flats
when his *boesem* friend, the AIDS activist Mike Matyeni, introduces
me to Vusumzi. He decides to share the intimate details of his love
life with me anonymously. "Vusumzi said he wanted to help other
men by telling his story," says Mike.

Rapidly, in a mixture of English and Cape Flats Afrikaans,
Vusumzi tells how as a teenager he moved with his mother to Cape
Town from his hometown, Lady Frere.

He was 13 years old when he saw his father's face for the first time, lying in a bed at the Red Cross Children's Hospital in Rondebosch. "I was burnt with boiling water and I couldn't walk. My dad brought me clothes in hospital, but I don't know how he knew my size."

As the youngest of five children, Vusumzi was his mother's pet. For his first two years in high school she sent him to a "coloured school" in Bonteheuwel. There he fell in love with Myra.

His dimples are etched deeper into his face. "We became serious. Saturdays Myra came to watch me play soccer and in the afternoons after school we had sex at a friend's house in Bonteheuwel. The relationship continued even when I went to a secondary school in Langa in Standard Eight."

In 1998 – his matric year – Myra summoned him to her home in Netreg, Bonteheuwel. He will never forget her words: "Vusumzi, I'm pregnant and I found out that I'm HIV positive."

He stirs his coffee faster and faster where he sits opposite me in a bustling café in town. In the wood-and-tin shack in his mother's backyard in Philippi on the Cape Flats, where he lives with his wife Elizabeth, "the walls have ears".

"I didn't say anything; but I knew I'd stay away," says Vusumzi softly. "Back at home I didn't feel like doing anything. All I could think was, I'm gonna die".

He started drinking heavily and refused to go to school. "I didn't know HIV could happen to me. I really trusted Myra."

To this day I am unable to get a straight answer from him about who brought the virus into the relationship. Vusumzi mostly alleges that he only "kissed" other girls while he was going out with Myra. Yet in an unguarded moment he uses the Xhosa expression *patla patla* (sex).

What really happened is impossible to know. Both his and Myra's memories had plunged into a black hole. All my attempts to accompany Vusumzi to see Myra had failed. Three times I met him at his home and three times he had conjured up a new excuse. The reason? Perhaps because *her* version of the story would cause him unbearable pain.

He describes how he had ignored Myra for six months after she tested positive for HIV. One day the then very pregnant 19-year-old eventually tracked him down to his mother's house in Philippi. Vusumzi sighs. "When I came home that night, my mother said: 'Your girlfriend is sleeping in your room, the one from Netreg you made pregnant'."

He still trembles when he recalls how Myra calmly instructed him that they should both tell his mother they are positive so that he could get help.

"I said to her: '*I'm* not positive, *you're* positive," says Vusumzi.

Myra's response? "I never had sex with anybody else but you."

That morning at five o'clock he ran away to his friends. When he eventually came home, he could tell Myra had confided to his mother. "My mom arranged for my older brother to take me to a private doctor on Monday to have me tested for HIV."

His worst fears were confirmed. "In front of my brother I said to the doctor: 'You're talking bullshit.' The doctor replied, 'Any other doctor will tell you the same thing – you are HIV positive.' I said, 'You will probably phone all the doctors in the Cape and tell them I'm positive before I go'."

The brothers went to two more doctors and Vusumzi kept shying away from the truth. When his and Myra's baby, Valerie, was born, Vusumzi's mother went to the maternity ward. "When my mom came back, she said: 'Vusumzi, you have a daughter.' I responded: 'It's not my child'."

His mother and sister continued visiting Myra and the baby on weekends. Vusumzi's family even invited the new mother and her baby to their home in Philippi for two weeks.

His eyes are dark. "I chased Myra and the child away."

He spills coffee on his neatly ironed shirt. "That's why Myra became a drug addict. Her mother asked me to go and talk to her and Myra said to me she would stop using if I drank my [antiretroviral] pills, otherwise I would die. I said 'No, I'm throwing the pills away'."

Soon after, he was admitted to Tygerberg Hospital with meningitis and a dangerously low CD4 count. Myra and little Valerie (at that time approximately two years old) visited him every day.

"One Sunday Myra and my family were there to visit and I saw them playing with the child as if it was their own. My brother said to me: 'It's not the child's fault that you have HIV, you have to accept your child'."

He clears his throat with a cough and lists the girls he had had sex with after leaving Myra. "No, no condoms. I thought it was not right that only I had the virus. Other girls needed to get it too."

He stares at the floor. "I thought that if you told women, they would spread stories about you. They wouldn't ask how you got it."

Sindiswa and Kolekile

The story of the women in his life reads like one long soap opera. In June 2001 Vusumzi met Sindiswa (27), "the love of his life" – a smart woman with an hourglass figure, who at the time was still at school.

Late in August he accompanied me to her small, bedless shack in the Kosovo squatter camp. Sindiswa recently moved there on her own after her five-year marriage with Thabo came to an end. "Thabo hit me and cheated on me," she says, her head held high.

Vusumzi is still head over heals for Sindiswa – even though the baby he had with his wife, Elizabeth, is only a couple of weeks old. He jokes around outside while Sindiswa tells me how Vusumzi started a relationship with her without him disclosing his status.

In December 2001 she fell pregnant with his child, and at four months she tested positive for HIV at the prenatal clinic.

"I immediately went to tell Vusumzi that I was positive." Sindiswa rolls her eyes. "He said we had to go for a test together to make sure that the results were correct. His test was also positive."

About a month later she found out from a friend that Vusumzi had known for a long time that he had the virus, but that he thought the whole thing was joke.

"I was angry; I was terribly hurt. I decided I had to leave."

Yet she couldn't "run away" from him. After Kolekile's birth, she forgave him. "I realised he was still the father of my son. In December 2003, Kolekile and I went to my mother in the Eastern Cape. I still had contact with Vusumzi then, but I knew it was over."

Later, on the phone, she tells me about all Vusumzi's other girl-friends – before and after Kolekile's birth. "I really loved him," she says softly, "but I gave him a second chance and he messed that up as well. He hasn't stopped apologising, but I only see him because of Kolekile."

That afternoon Vusumzi looks pale.

"I loved Sindiswa so much – I did not want to lose her. That is why I didn't tell her about the HIV. The fight only started when she found out that she was HIV positive and that I had known about the HIV. Every time I saw her she was in pain. I couldn't handle it."

He is riddled by remorse. "When she took me back I had another girlfriend. Later I couldn't even look at Sindiswa. I said to her she just had to go."

Lindiwe and Maria

The mother of Vusumzi's third child, Maria (5), is an HIV-positive woman, Lindiwe, who he met during a march of the Treatment Action Campaign. "She fell pregnant within a month," he says. "We broke up because she was too jealous of my other girls."

This time Vusumzi's mother put her foot down and ordered her youngest son to stop "playing around" and tie the knot. Meanwhile he got word that an ex-girlfriend in the Eastern Cape had fallen ill. There's another one in the Cape he's too afraid to see.

He speaks softly. "If I were to find out today that the one in the Cape is also ill, I would hide my eyes and close my ears. Back then I felt nothing, but as life went on I started to realise that it was wrong. That is why I decided in December to pay *lobola* to Elizabeth's family."

Elizabeth and Zolani

On a chilly spring day I meet Elizabeth, Vusumzi's beautiful but withdrawn wife. While he takes a trolley down the street to the neighbours to fetch water, she breastfeeds their baby, Zolani. "I saw Vusumzi around in the community here and I recognised that he was a good man; the right man. The baby is healthy and we are happy," she says absently.

Elizabeth discovered in 2007 that she was HIV positive. When she started going steady with Vusumzi two years later, she initially hid her status from him. "I loved him and thought that he would run away."

She looks down. "I heard in the community that Vusumzi was positive, but we only disclosed to each other when he asked me to marry him. He supported me. We go to the clinic together and he takes his medicine."

Later Vusumzi says Elizabeth still does not want people to know about the virus. "I said to her the secrets would eat her up from the inside. When she sits at home and says nothing for three days I get worried. What if she's in pain, maybe she's thinking of killing herself?"

He smiles proudly, a "new" man. "You can ask Mike Matyeni – I go all over the place – to Kraaifontein, Worcester, Robertson, De Doorns, Ceres, and I tell people I'm HIV positive."

"Please forgive me"

Spring is in full bloom when I meet Vusumzi again in a café in town. He drinks one beer after the other, desperately clutching at the bottle. At last he confesses: "Elizabeth wants to take the baby and go to the Eastern Cape. I think she wants to leave me. She doesn't trust me with other women, but I don't sleep around any more."

Does he want to save his marriage?

He hesitates. "If I could make one thing right, I would go to Sindiswa's mother and ask for forgiveness. I gave the virus to her daughter. Sindiswa is still my number one."

He reconsiders, suddenly rudderless. "But if Elizabeth decides she wants to stay, I will forget about Sindiswa. It's my duty; I married her."

This is to be my last meeting with Vusumzi and muddled thoughts run through my head: He grew up in an era of AIDS denial; he's one of millions robbed of his manhood by poverty. Above all: AIDS is not a story of "guilty" or "not guilty".

Cautiously I direct the conversation towards his four children from four different mothers – all of them HIV negative, according to him. The past few months he had had very little contact with them. He does not pay maintenance, and he has not told any of their mothers that since August he had been working at a factory earning R110 a day.

"The pain in my heart is that I have a small baby that I see every day. Then I think: Have the others got anything to eat? What are they doing? That is why I have to sort out my life. I don't know what their mothers think of me."

He grows pensive. "I feel guilty about Myra and Sindiswa – especially Sindiswa. And I keep thinking about my mother. I don't think she trusts me any more and she did everything for me. I always say to them: 'I did something wrong – please forgive me'."

His eyes meet mine, then he lowers his forehead. "The more I run away, the more I hurt people. I couldn't face the truth – that was the reason. Now I want to stay in one place."

He greets, finishes his beer and walks away. He starts jogging, then running through the city rush – away from his story and away from himself.

Some names have been changed. Originally published in Afrikaans as "Geheime maak seer" on 20 November 2010 in By, *a supplement in* Die Burger, Volksblad *and* Beeld.

"Saveth me from death"

Willemien Brümmer

Not all men run away when HIV comes to stay. Lester Karolus told Willemien Brümmer how he "became a travelling circus" when his wife fell ill.

"I'm mommy *and* daddy in this shack," says Lester Karolus (55) and winks proudly. "My wife can't get up. I'm her mother and *ma* for the kids as well."

Lester is a hardened man with a scarred face. His hands are enormous; his wiry body muscular. His Afrikaans is the poetry of the streets. In his younger days he was *deurmekaar* – "in and out of prison".

His face, brayed by poverty, becomes almost devout. "They say the older you get, the more you learn. When I decided to get married, I became a new man."

His shack or *hok*, as he calls it, is a wooden hut three by six metres in his sister's backyard in Manenberg on the Cape Flats. Inside it smells of disease and urine. Outside in the street the women sit on the *skinnerbankies* (gossip benches). Groups of adolescents groove about. This is gangster area – the playground of the Hard Livings, the Americans, the Clever Kids, the Jesters.

Lester shrugs. "We stay in a messy place, but that's not our line. Often the gangsters shoot at each other in the street; we just dodge the bullets."

Manenberg's notorious gangs are, after all, the least of his problems. Next to him on the unmade single bed sit his sons Richard (12) and Lester Junior (7). They are skinny and their noses are runny. His wife Katy (50) is in the single bed opposite him, a whispering bundle of bones.

It is July and everything outside is muddy. Katy, who has been waiting "for a council house for 22 years", coughs. "It is cold in here and it's cold outside. When it rains, the water runs into our shack."

Lester nods. "At this time of the month we are hungry. But we have *pap* and bread and a teabag and sugar. What I really am after is for the kids to eat healthy. They can't take their pills on an empty stomach."

"My wife's right hand"

My first encounter with Lester is in April at the paediatric AIDS Unit at Groote Schuur Hospital. He is the only dad in the bustling unit. He is a lone man in a sea of women – mothers with their children, grandmothers, caregivers, doctors, nurses. A smiling counsellor introduces Lester to me. "He's one of the few men who stayed when he found out that his wife was HIV positive. We think he is negative."

Lester is friendly, he likes to talk, but he insists on calling me "Missus". "You see, Missus, it's for *them* that I'm here," he says, pointing at his kids. "My wife became sick first, and then we took tests that said Richard and Lester Junior were born positive, but I'm clear. My mission here is to get the medication."

He hesitates. "I knew nothing about HIV before. Sweet blow all, Missus. But I'm my wife's right hand – even now. I became a travelling circus – from GF Jooste to Lentegeur, to Tygerberg. I spent many nights there."

He shakes his head. "I know many men who left their wives and kids just like that because of the sickness, but I think they just wanted a reason to get away. I thought I'll just carry on with my burden. This is the cross I have to bear – and it's a cast-iron cross, you know."

He tells me how he had to stop working last year to look after his wife and children. At the moment he works for minimal pay as a "permanent casual" at an oil-drilling company.

"I didn't know how important it was, but my wife stopped the medication for eight months. Last year August she came back to the hospital for the first time. She couldn't walk, she didn't eat, she was so thin."

He bows his head.

"There's a woman in our street – if she sees Katy she sings a hymn: '*Haal my uit die dode en sit my in die lewe*' [Saveth me from death and bring me back to life]. Many people have prayed for her, but it's through God's grace that she came to life again."

"I'm made of skin and bones"

Lester's story starts in 1955 in Claremont, Cape Town, as the fourth youngest of 14 children – before the forced removals. Initially his mother was working in a white woman's house. His father drove the *nagwa*, a horse-drawn carriage that went to replace the buckets in people's lavatories. At 13, in Standard Four, Lester's dad took him out of school to get him to start working in a furniture factory in Lansdowne.

"The way I'm struggling now, my dad also struggled. My mom was a very sickly woman. She had this vinegar rag with potatoes that she cut open and held against her head for the pain. My dad said from now on *he* works with the money, *he* will make the food."

His face is contorted with laughter as he remembers how his dad balanced bags of vegetables and meat that he bought from the hawkers and the butchery on his bike. "My ma never needed to worry about anything. He ran everything in the house. When he made food at night, he would scratch the pot so hard you had to hear there were no second helpings. He knew what to do, he was organised, Missus."

He smiles. "Nowadays I tell my youngest sister I've become like my dad. But I don't mind, I'll do it, it suits me. After all, I've got my dad's name."

As a teenager, after his mother's stroke, Lester had to be "her legs". "My ma was fat, but I carried her with these two hands, never letting her fall. From the car to the toilet, to the people she wanted to see. It was only after her death that I felt like getting a wife."

At 23, Lester married his first wife, Gadidja, with whom he had eight children. Her family was Muslim – "big-time hawkers" – and he gutted and sold fish for them. "We had a long and difficult marriage. Gadidja was spiteful, she wasn't used to the hard life; her family was quite thick in cash."

Ten years ago, shortly after Gadidja and Lester were divorced in a court of law, Gadidja died in her five-roomed house in Manenberg. Somewhat embarrassed, he says: "I was quite terrible that time; I was going with Katy then."

He musters a sly smile. "I met Katy on the streets of Manenberg, then I asked her out on a date. She's a make-believer. I thought the things in her mouth were rubies, but I later found out she'd put nail polish on her teeth."

At the time she already had a daughter (now 23) and a son (now 16) with other men. Her last boyfriend, a member of the Hard Livings gang, was serving a 15-year prison sentence.

"When Katy and I got together, our son Richard (now 12) came very soon after," says Lester. "I was straight with Katy: 'If you don't want me, talk to me. I don't want to skip from woman to woman any more.'"

He beams with joy. "She wanted me. We are meant for each another, Missus."

They got married in his sister's house in Manenberg, after Katy had been discharged from hospital for the umpteenth time. While she was ill, the children stayed with Katy's sister-in-law, Auntie Dollie.

Lester's face growns dark. "Auntie Dollie wanted to take the kids from me. She wanted to go to the social workers, but I put the brakes on that one. We got married especially so that no one could take the kids away. So I made it legal, written on paper."

He clenches his enormous hands into fists. "But I can't depend on Katy, Missus. Now I have to take her place, fill her shoes." He sighs. "You see, Missus, I'm made of skin and bones. You don't want to borrow every day while you wait for Friday, for payday. When I get home tonight, there's no food for the pot. She doesn't even try to make an effort, she can't."

Proudly he tells me how he gives Richard and Lester Junior their pills at seven o'clock each evening. In the morning, before he walks to the station, he leaves Katy and the children's pills each in their own little pile.

"Maybe it's the illness that makes Katy forget, I don't know. Sometimes when I'm at work I think that woman has gone to the hospital today with those two children. And then I start worrying: Does she hold their hands when they cross the street? The little one is wild. And then, when I get home, I see she hasn't even gone to fetch the pills. The next day I have to get into the taxi myself, because they *must* have the pills, Missus." He rolls his eyes. "You don't hear those children say: 'Mommy this, Mommy that.' When they come in the door, it's 'Daddy, I'm hungry'."

"He wasn't angry"

On a Saturday at the end of October I get the chance to talk to Katy alone for the first time. She's skeletal, her voice hardly above a whisper. She hasn't washed for some time and the skin around her mouth is a raw, dry crust.

We sit in my car some distance from their shack in Manenberg. "Tomorrow everybody will be talking about me again," she says and closes the window.

I clear my throat. "Your hospital records show that yet again you haven't picked up your pills each month."

Her eyes are dead.

"Last month I didn't take the pills, they made me throw up. I gave the children their pills in the morning and Lester gives it to them at night when he comes home from work."

It has only been since her last hospital visit four days ago that she has attempted to take the pills again. "The counsellor said I had to take it, otherwise I won't be seeing my kids for much longer."

How long has she known she has the virus?

She doesn't answer for some time. Then: "When Richard [12] was still a baby, he was lying at the Red Cross Hospital with HIV," she admits. "They explained to me what HIV was and they took my blood. They saw I also have it."

She looks down. "I was ashamed to tell Lester. In hospital the nurses talked about HIV openly when Richard and Lester Junior had to go to hospital for TB, but he was too stupid to notice. I tried to hide our HIV. I thought he would leave me with the two kids." She attempts a smile. "But I think he accepted it even before I told him. Luckily he wasn't angry, he was friendly."

"A lifelong something"

Soon after, I meet Lester and Richard at a sunny café next to a park in town. Lester is thinner, his face more angular than before. It is springtime, but he has a persistent cough.

"Are you sick?" I ask.

His voice is gruff.

"I've got my hands full, Missus. I'm tired, my wife's not helping much. I try to understand, but I'm finished, *klaar*. This time of the year I'm even more aware of her illness. I can see it when her eyes go wild..."

When did he last have a test?

"Last year I went in the sixth month, and it was clear."

Silence. "But I must go again. I know there is a chance I might get it, but there's a whole container full of condoms in our room. Richard and I sleep on one bed and Katy and the other two [Lester Junior and Katy's own 16 year old] sleep on the other bed. We're not really in line for sex and those things any more."

Does he ever talk to Katy and the kids about dying?

He stays mute for seconds. "Ja, I talk to them – especially when that insurance thing comes on TV – those death benefits. Then I say to Katy: 'I don't like it, they just say we're all going to die'; I *know* we're going to die."

He sighs. "It's not as if I don't worry, Missus, but I can't let Katy see I'm worried. I must stay calm; I just pretend everything is okay."

Richard tiptoes a little closer. He looks small for a 12 year old. He insists on calling me "doctor".

Carefully I ask: "Richard, do you take your pills every day?"

He talks softly. "My dad said I must take my pills every day, now I do it every day, doctor. There have been a few times that I didn't take it, I don't know for how long. Ja, doctor, I became ill. My ma lies in bed, she's not taking her pills every day. Then she becomes angry, doctor. I don't know why, doctor."

He sniffles and drops his head on his knees. "I'm also angry, doctor. I'm scared that something will happen to her."

"Does your mom look after you when your dad goes to work?"

"My mom gives us *pap* in the morning and then she sits in the sun. When she's finished with that, she puts the music on and sings along with the music. No, doctor, she doesn't play with us."

He starts crying and shifts a little closer to his father. "My daddy looks after me, doctor. When my dad comes home, my ma doesn't get up."

"Do you know what illness you have?"

"Ja, doctor, my daddy said the doctor said I have HIV," he says through his blocked nose. "But I don't know what that is."

Lester sits down behind him, whispers in his ear. "That's the sickness the doctor said you have. You're going to grow up with the pills, it's for life, this thing. One day you will walk the road alone. You listen to what Daddy is telling you."

Lester turns to me as if he is expecting the question. "Even though it's hard at the moment, I'll never leave Katy – never. Until death do us part … I love my kids. I can't give up now. I've made my bed."

Names have been changed. Originally published in Afrikaans as "Haal my uit die dode" on 27 November 2010 in By, *a supplement in* Die Burger, Volksblad *and* Beeld.

In the winter of 2010, Nardus Engelbrecht accompanied journalist Willemien Brümmer on her expeditions to informal settlements outside Cape Town. In this photo essay Engelbrecht's images capture the daily struggles of dedicated father and husband Lester as they play out against a bleak landscape characterised by disease and poverty.

Without identifying the subjects, Engelbrecht manages to pin down the experience of a man doing everything he can to keep his ailing HIV-positive wife and their two HIV-positive sons afloat.

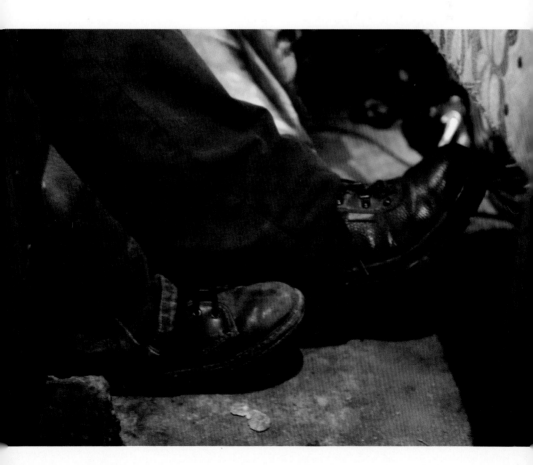

Proudly, Lester tells me how he gives Richard and Lester Junior their pills at seven o'clock each evening. In the morning, before he walks to the station, he leaves Katy and the children's pills each in their own little pile wrapped in toilet paper.

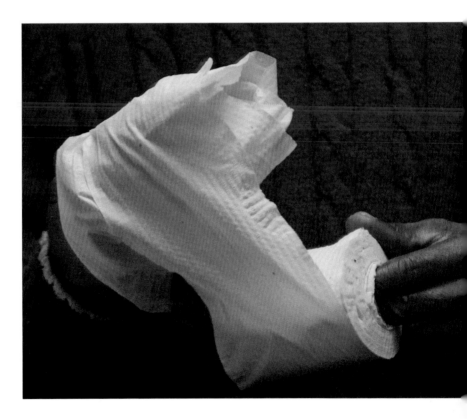

"When I get home from work, I see she [my wife] hasn't even gone to fetch the pills. The next day I have to get into the taxi myself, because they must have the pills, Missus."

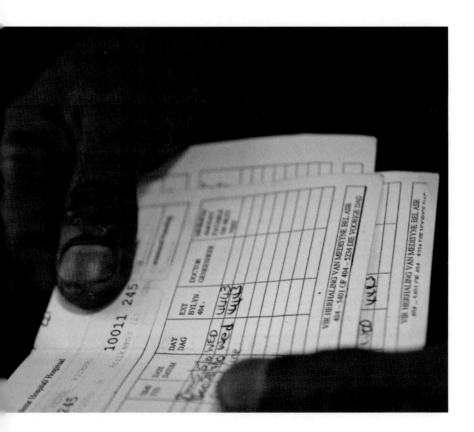

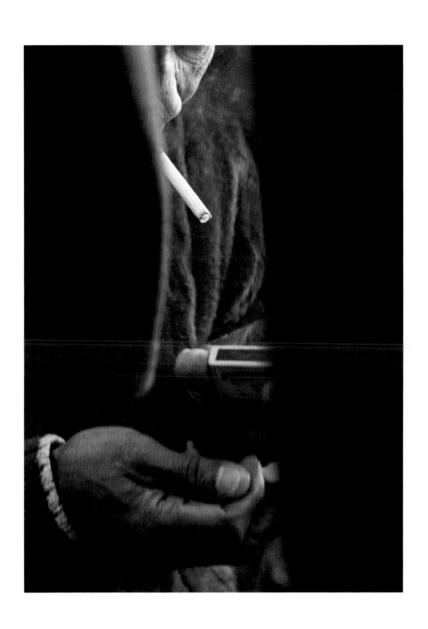

"We stay in a messy place, but that's not our line. Often gangsters shoot at each other in the street; we just dodge the bullets."

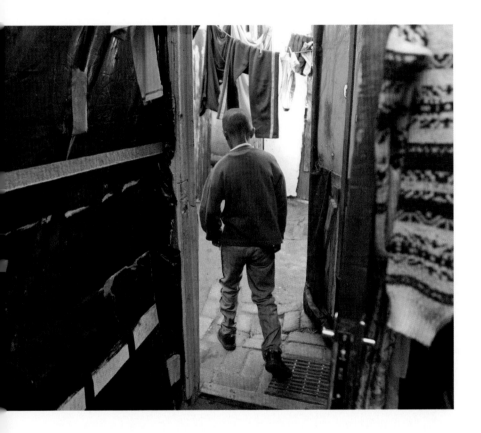

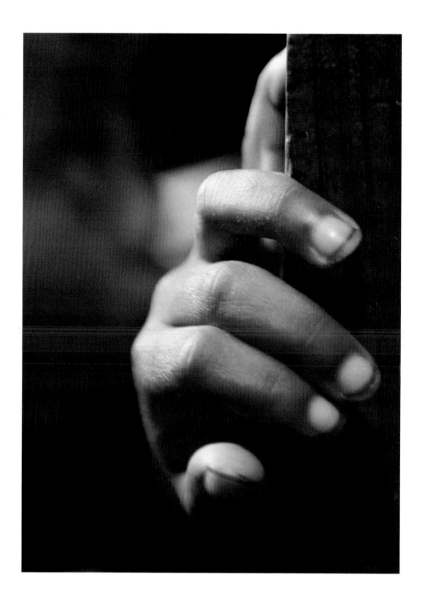

"HIV is the sickness the doctor said you have. You're going to grow up with the pills, it's for life, this thing. One day you will walk the road alone. You listen to what Daddy is telling you."

"I know men who left their wives and kids just like that because of the sickness, but I think they just wanted a reason to get away. Then I think I'll just carry on with my burden. This is the cross I have to bear – and it's a cast-iron cross, you know."

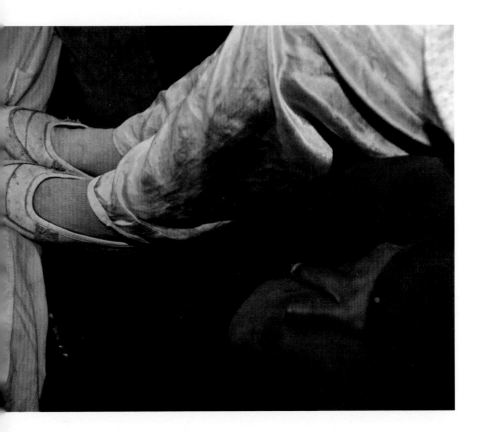

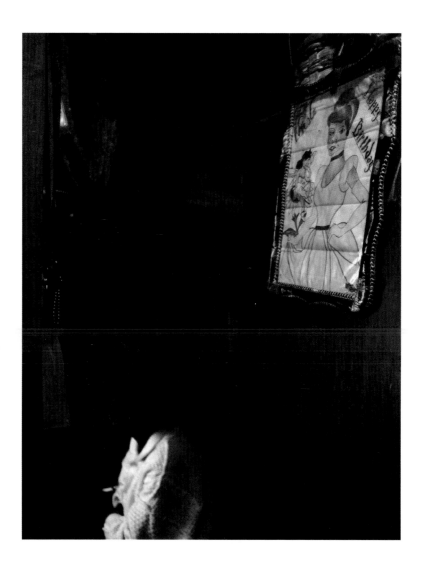

"I met Katy on the streets of Manenberg, then I asked her out on a date. She's a make-believer. I thought the things in her mouth were rubies, but I later found out she'd put nail polish on her teeth."

Fathers & partners

"I didn't understand why my wife insisted on not breast-feeding. I asked her, and she told me that that was the choice she made at the clinic."

"My father was a ladies' man. He had plenty of girlfriends. He liked them young too."

Fathers & partners / Introduction

The project's junior journalism fellows Lungi Langa and Thabisile Dlamini both made men as fathers their focus during their tenure with the HIV & AIDS Media Project's fellowship programme. In 2009 and 2010 they met a number of men from all walks of life and sketched a varied account of the different faces of fatherhood in South Africa. Their coverage of men as fathers defies simple hero-dad or bad-dad dichotomies and instead presents readers with fatherhood in all its complexity.

Traditional notions of masculinity dictate that family men should be independent protectors and breadwinners, and that nurturing, caring and home-cooked meals are better left up to their female foil.[1] But this cool and aloof father does not cut it any more. Men's lack of involvement as partners in pregnancy and later as fathers has been fingered as a serious limitation confronting their own health and that of their families.

Where parenthood in the context of HIV is concerned, the stakes are much higher. Uninvolved fathers present a missed opportunity to encourage men to take responsibility for their own health and that of their families. It is also a missed chance to debunk misconceptions around gendered roles in health care. This is particularly evident in the prevention of mother-to-child transmission (PMTCT) of HIV where the emphasis tends to be exclusively on mothers, often to the detriment of their partners.

This is the case for Eliot in Langa's "Daddies in the dark". Despite his best intentions to be part of his wife's pregnancy, Eliot is consistently left out of the loop. As a result, he is oblivious to his wife's HIV-positive status and her participation in the PMTCT programme. This leaves him baffled by her decision to bottle feed, and places him

1   Connell (1992).

in poor stead to properly care for his new child.[2] This secrecy also endangers his own health as Eliot remains unaware that he too might be HIV positive. Like Eliot, Sabelo, who is featured in the same story, was also kept in the dark. After his wife's death from pneumonia and the subsequent discovery that he too is HIV positive, Sabelo is left to piece together the puzzle to explain why and how his 11-year-old son is HIV negative.

Langa's journalism makes a strong case for the inclusion of fathers in prenatal and postnatal care. Men who are welcomed into PMTCT programmes are more likely to know and accept their female partner's status. Because they are more knowledgeable, they can also support their partners in making decisions and ensure that PMTCT strategies such as antiretroviral treatment (ART) and infant feeding are implemented.[3] These men are usually more likely to go with their partners to antenatal clinic visits and test for HIV.[4]

For both Eliot and Sabelo, it is their partner's failure to disclose that keeps them ignorant. Langa's journalism, however, reserves judgement. Instead, her coverage remains mindful of how these women's fear of discrimination, physical violence, accusations of infidelity and abandonment often feed into secrecy.[5]

But a partner's silence is not the only barrier to men's involvement. Sabelo, like many other South African men, is not afforded the luxury of family or paternity leave to accompany his partner to her antenatal visits. Moreover, the predominantly female world of

---

2　At the time the journalism was produced, government policy advocated for exclusive bottle-feeding to minimise the risk of transferring HIV to the baby. By the time this book went to press, policy had been amended to instead advocate for exclusive breastfeeding, provided both mother and baby are taking ART.

3　Tijou Traoré, Querre, Brou, Leroy, Desclaux and Desgrées-du-Loû (2009).

4　Theuring, Nchimbi, Jordan-Harder and Harms (2010).

5　Medley, Garcia-Moreno, McGill and Maman (2004).

PMTCT and health care in general means men often receive a less than warm welcome at clinics and other public health spaces. As a result, even if men are able to attend these visits, like Eliot, they may be asked to wait outside.

Langa's second article provides a blend of science and personal narrative that breathes life into normally stale coverage of conception among HIV-positive parents.

In "Fathering hope", Langa introduces men who tread the long road from coming to terms with their HIV status all the way to fatherhood, driving home the message that living with HIV does not mean having to shut the door on being a father.

Studies have shown that HIV-positive men long to become fathers, citing fatherhood as a role that gives them renewed purpose in life.[6] For some HIV-positive parents, having children also serves as a means of reinforcing their own identity and social standing.[7] Yet HIV-related stigma and prejudice remain formidable barriers for couples living with HIV who want to conceive, with many anticipating disapproval from healthcare staff.[8]

Refreshingly, the stories of Andile and Gcobani not only highlight the medical techniques that allow people living with HIV to have children, but also tackle the reality of stigma and discrimination that continue to drive people with HIV to desperate and dangerous lengths.

But fatherhood does not stop with conception, pregnancy and birth. Raising children in the context of HIV has received even less attention than men's roles as partners in the PMTCT process.[9] In

---

6   Sherr and Barry (2004).

7   Cooper, Harries, Myer, Orner and Bracken (2007).

8   Paiva, Filipe, Santos, Lima and Segurado (2003).

9   Morrell and Richter (2006) distinguish between fathers and fatherhood, stating that fathering a child in the biological sense does not automatically mean that men take

South Africa discussions around fathers have largely centred round the crisis facing fatherhood.[10] Dismal reports paint a picture of a legion of absent dads or fathers who were present but were less than stellar. Despite there being clear connections, not much of this has been discussed in the context of HIV.

In her four-part series on fathers, Dlamini undertook to change this. With carefully crafted vignettes of fatherhood and family life as played out in a world of HIV, these stories get to grips with a set of deeply complex issues, including testing, treatment and disclosure. Importantly, Dlamini's journalism teases out how ideals of the "real man" sometimes compromise men's ability to be great dads.

The first narrative in her series is delivered through the eyes of a daughter in her early twenties who must endure a tumultuous relationship with an abusive and unsupportive father who is often ill but refuses to acknowledge that he might have HIV. This heart-rending account touches on a variety of issues central to the epidemic, including multiple and concurrent partners, traditional medicine, intergenerational sex and HIV denialism.

In the second story, a teenaged Lerato welcomes back a father whom she has never known and who was not a part of her life largely because he could not provide for his family. This is an all-too-familiar scenario where men's inability to do the things that "real men" do, such as provide for and protect their families, results in feelings of powerlessness and shame, which ultimately drive them to abandon their families.[11]

on fatherhood as a role. Conversely men who are not the biological fathers (e.g. stepfathers) of children sometimes take on the fatherhood role in relation to those children.

10   Morrell and Richter (2006).

11   Ramphele and Richter (2006).

Lerato also discovers that her father is HIV positive. Dlamini then traverses a terrain only occasionally covered in the media: parents' disclosure of their HIV-positive status to their children. A European study concluded that HIV-affected children experience more emotional and behavioural problems, but that this could be remedied by making HIV services more family oriented.[12] The journalism reflects this, as a troubled Lerato nearly fails her eighth school year. Ultimately, though still anxious about not having enough time with him, Lerato's reunion with her father plays out well for both.

The third story again ties into how poverty and traditional masculinity affect men's ability to be good all-round fathers, albeit with a bit of a twist. Mandla's story spotlights how sickness affects men's perceptions of themselves and their ability to be "good" fathers. Because HIV gets in the way of working and providing, it often leaves men feeling ashamed and emasculated.[13] Mandla's statement that, after being diagnosed with HIV, he "didn't feel worthy" agrees with this disjuncture between illness and dominant masculinity.

In Mandla's sub-narrative covering his relationship with his own father, HIV-denialism among men rears its head again. Against the backdrop of South Africa circa 1997, when myths, controversy and taboos festered, like his father, Mandla refuses to believe that HIV exists, claiming it is a "white man's disease".[14]

The last piece in Dlamini's arsenal is about the "all-around father". But Dlamini certainly does not mean this in the sense that the key character, Nhlanhla Mavundla, is being a good all-rounder when it comes to fatherhood. Rather, Nhlanhla, an HIV-positive activist, "gets around" – having two families with two different

12   Nöstlinger, Bartoli, Gordillo, Roberfroid and Colebunders (2006).

13   Courtenay (2000).

14   Fourie and Meyer (2010).

women. This results in Nhlanhla's children not getting the full benefit of their father's emotional support and attention. Yet he feels that decking his kids out in Nike and buying them fast food, makes up for that. Again the emphasis is on the masculine ideals of economic support and provision as the role of the father, while nurturing and emotional support fall by the wayside.

Openly HIV positive, Nhlanhla's story is a far cry from the other men's stories of HIV-denialism. But it does alert readers to the equally problematic matter of the fissure that often separates knowledge and behaviour – where people continue to have unprotected sex with multiple partners despite their HIV-positive status. Again, some of the blame can be apportioned to rigid ideas of what it means to be a man, leading Nhlanhla to believe that he needs to prove his masculinity by continuing to philander.

Media images of fathers and partners

A total of 74 articles were returned through searches using keywords related to conception, HIV, PMTCT, fathers and fatherhood. Given the limited coverage on fathers in the HIV & AIDS Media Project's specialised HIV-related media databases, additional keyword searches were conducted using the IOL, SowetanLIVE and TimesLIVE websites.[15] The coverage yielded from the searches could be divided into three broad categories: HIV and conception; PMTCT-related coverage; and fathers and fatherhood.

In our analysis, media coverage of fathers and partners in the context of HIV is conspicuously absent. Given that a staggering 5.6 million South Africans are living with HIV, this is disconcerting. Pregnancy and conception in the context of HIV do make headlines,

---

15 These websites span a multitude of publications, which include *The Star, Sunday Independent, The Saturday Star, The Times, Sunday World, Sowetan* and *The Sunday Times.*

but fathers are nowhere to be found. Fathers, on the other hand, are in the news, though never in relation to HIV. When fathers are covered, they are placed into one of two categories: failed man or hero. Both draw heavily on traditional ideas of what makes a man, "a man". The omission of men and their extremely stereotypical treatment where they are mentioned does not bode well for South Africa's existing crisis in fatherhood.

Our analysis also revealed a pattern over time, where coverage of fathers begins with conception, dropping off during pregnancy, only to pick up again in the postnatal stage of the child's life. The result is a great "no-man's land" that stretches through pregnancy and infancy. The glaring absence of men in these stages can be linked to society's understanding of what it means to be a "real" man. Coverage of conception is consistent with traditional ideas of masculinity because it fits with ideas of man's virility and sexual potency. Tying men to pregnancy and care for babies and small children is out of the question because these activities are too soft and nurturing and cross the line of what a "real" man does.

Ladies first: Men as partners in the South African media

In our analysis, while the media's engagement with HIV and conception was already lamentably slim, with only three articles dedicated to the matter, most of the coverage focused on the medical aspects of having a baby when one or both partners is living with HIV.[16,17,18] In this rather technical landscape, there was one piece of narrative journalism that focused on an HIV-positive man's journey from accept-

16   Sedibe, D. "Pregnancy guidelines for HIV+ couples", *The Star* (June 2011).

17   Khoaele, K. "Finding love and healing", *Move!* (August 2011).

18   "New hope for childless HIV-positive couples", *The Star* (April 2011).

ing his status and taking steps to stay healthy to reconciling with his
HIV-negative partner and then their efforts to have a child together.[19]

But all is not rosy. The piece explains how the couple conceived,
and then confirms that mother and child are both negative but skips
over pregnancy altogether. Even the small fact box on PMTCT that
accompanies the article is "mum" on the role of dads, repeatedly mentioning "moms" and "the mom's doctor". It is the same dad-shaped
hole that appears to characterise most coverage on pregnancy and
PMTCT.

The second category consisted of 13 PMTCT-related articles.
These were a mix of narratives and news reports. Much like the
coverage of conception, news reports on pregnancy and PMTCT in
particular focused on the need for, or the efficacy of, medical interventions such as ART.[20,21,22,23] Even the sole feature article on maternal health and HIV did not suggest that male partners' involvement
in PMTCT (and pregnancy in general) might improve the health of
mothers or of their babies.[24]

A piece of narrative journalism that appeared in *The Times* on
World AIDS Day was the only promising story to come out of the
PMTCT coverage.[25] The article sensitively detailed the experiences
of a mother-to-be undergoing PMTCT to protect her unborn child
from the virus. The piece makes multiple mentions of the woman's
boyfriend, who often is not there to support her because he "lives

19 Khoaele, K. "Finding love and healing", *Move!* (August 2011).

20 Majavu, A. "New targets set for health", *The Times* (November 2011).

21 AFP. "HIV prevention in babies '96% successful'", *The New Age* (June 2011).

22 Majavu, A. "Hike ARV access to expectant moms", *Sowetan* (November 2011).

23 Sapa. "HIV rises among pregnant women", *Sowetan* (November 2011).

24 Makhanya, C. "Pregnancy and your health", *Daily Sun* (February 2012).

25 McLea, H. "Thanks to God for Nevirapine", *The Times* (December 2011).

and works far away". This is the same reason why he misses the birth of their child. Although it is not in the scope of the piece to explore and interrogate men's role in PMTCT, it does shed light on some of the barriers to men's involvement in the context of extreme poverty and migrant labour.

Proof that men can and should be involved beyond conception comes in the form of a Brothers for Life advertisement that appeared in the *Daily Sun* during our period of analysis.[26,27] The full-page advert directed at men explains the details of PMTCT and how fathers can get involved. While the piece does not constitute coverage of fathers and their partners, it does demonstrate that it is possible to produce engaging and informative coverage on men in reproductive and maternal health.

Saints or sinners: Fathers in the South African media

While there was some media coverage on men conceiving children in the context of HIV, in our analysis media coverage on fatherhood in the context of HIV was virtually non-existent. Outside of HIV, fathers do, however, make headlines. We thus extended our analysis to include images of fathers in the media in a more general sense. All in all, 58 articles were returned through searches related to fathers and fatherhood.

The most common theme in our assessment was fathers as perpetrators of violence. An overwhelming 33 articles centred on fathers directing their violent behaviour towards their own families, mainly children and spouses. In these articles fathers were responsible for

---

26 Brothers for Life is an organisation that targets men in South Africa, promoting healthier behaviours and addressing issues such as gender-based violence, condom use and HIV testing.

27 Brothers for Life adevrtisement. *What is PMTCT?* in *Daily Sun* (August 2011).

everything from negligence and kidnapping to rape, family murder-suicide and brutally attacking and killing their own children.[28,29,30,31] In only a small number of articles were fathers the victims of violence.

While many of the reports on violent fathers did not get into much detail, in most cases the fathers were conveyed as "deadbeat dads", men who had a "questionable" history, such as owning fire-arms and taking drugs. These articles seemed to convey the implicit message – "They should have seen it coming" – and that bad men do not make good dads. Some articles did buck the trend of simplistic portraits of "bad" dads, painting a more complex picture where dads who commit acts of violence are not always the clear, archetypal villain.[32] These reports left behind the black-and-white, saint-or-sinner dichotomies created by the rest of the media coverage, offering more dynamic and harder-to-swallow portraits of seemingly good men who do bad things.

The second major theme in the analysis stands in complete contrast to that of fathers as perpetrators of violence, namely fathers as heroes. With only six articles falling into this subcategory, there were not nearly as many of these articles as there were on violent and dangerous dads. But the complete opposition of the two themes is important in illustrating the "either-or" split that seems to characterise coverage on fathers.

Related to the coverage on fathers as heroes was a small group of articles that saw fathers appealing or advocating on behalf of their children. The five articles within this group ranged from fathers

28   Nombembe, P. "Remorseful dad faces the music", *www.timeslive.co.za* (February 2012).

29   Sapa. "Eastern Cape Dad allegedly kidnaps, rapes daughter", *www.timeslive.co.za* (October 2011).

30   Sapa. "Dad throws baby against wall", *www.sowetanlive.co.za* (June 2011).

31   Omar, Y. "Bloody suburban house of horror", *www.iol.co.za* (January 2012).

32   Dolley, C. "The quiet man who lived a life of crime", *www.iol.co.za* (December 2011).

appealing for help locating their missing children to a father going to court to secure funds for surgery for his young son.

Of the coverage that portrayed dads as heroes, fathers sacrificing themselves to protect their children was a major theme.[33] In contrast to their violent counterparts, all of these men were represented as hardworking. Particularly illustrative of this is the story of a "father of five" killed on the job during the Cape Flats bread war. The article framed the event as the tragic loss of a breadwinner who is "a responsible family man".

Celebrity-based coverage also followed the "deadbeat dad" versus "good hero dad" trend. Four of the six articles within this category focused on "bad" dads.[34,35,36] Some of these were reconciliatory stories, with adult children expressing the desire to forgive their fathers. This included an article on American singer Kelly Rowland who wants to "forgive" her father whose drinking problem drove her mother away.[37]

Two stories on celebrities following in their role-model fathers' footsteps were the foil for celeb stories on "deadbeat" dads. These stories featured local up-and-coming stars Roboshane Lekoelea and Nonkululeko Dube and how they drew inspiration from their dads, soccer star Steve Lekoelea[38] and musician Lucky Dube respectively.[39]

33 Skade, T. "Heroic dad dies with triplets", *www.iol.co.za* (March 2011).

34 Mahlangu, B. "Miss SA Teen wants nothing to do with dad", *www.sowetanlive.co.za* (January 2012).

35 Makhubele, M. "This is for you, Dad", *www.timeslive.co.za* (June 2011).

36 Bang showbiz. "Jay-Z scarred by father", *www.sowetanlive.co.za* (November 2011).

37 Bang showbiz. "She last saw her dad when she was 7", *www.sowetanlive.co.za* (November 2011).

38 Moholoa, R. "Lekoelea follows in dad's footsteps", *www.sowetanlive.co.za* (October 2011).

39 Sibiya, G. "Dube in dad's steps to fame", *www.sowetanlive.co.za* (June 2011).

Other than these "star power" stories, coverage of the crisis of fatherhood was thin, with only four articles addressing this pressing issue.[40,41,42,43] While there was a small sample of articles covering the impact that absent fathers had on children, these were largely topical pieces driven by the release of a report by the South African Institute of Race Relations.[44] Surprisingly, very few articles covered the related issues of custody and child maintenance.[45,46]

The crisis of fatherhood facing South Africa is a result of a complex web of interwoven factors. Poverty and migrancy springing from South Africa's turbulent history exacerbate the often unachievable ideals of dominant masculinity. But the power to facilitate change lies within the reach of the media. Considered, balanced media coverage can help make alternative emancipatory masculinities available to men through actively and consciously rewriting masculine roles and repertoires. Offering up alternative ways of being a man opens up the space for men to become emotionally available, supportive partners and fathers who take an interest in their own health and the health of their loved ones.

40   Pakade, N. "Role of Dads must be reinforced", *Sowetan* (April 2011).

41   Sonile, N. "Fathers not to be ignored', *The Citizen* (June 2011).

42   Ledwaba, L. "A dadless, angry generation", *City Press* (April 2011).

43   Sowetan editorial. "Absent fathers", *www.sowetanlive.co.za* (April 2011).

44   South African Institute of Race Relations. (2011) *First steps to healing the South African family.*

45   IOL. "Lobola dad to get kids", *www.iol.co.za* (March 2011).

46   Nombembe, P. "Runaway parents in big trouble", *www.timeslive.co.za* (December 2011).

References /

Cooper, D; Harries, J; Myer, L; Orner, P; and Bracken, H. (2007) "'Life is still going on': Reproductive intentions among HIV-positive women and men in South Africa." *Social Science & Medicine*, 65 (2), 274–283.

Courtenay, W. (2000) "Constructions of masculinity and their influence on men's well-being: A theory of gender and health." *Social Science & Medicine*, 50, 1385–1401.

Medley, A; Garcia-Moreno, C; McGill, S; and Maman, S. (2004) "Rates, barriers and outcomes of HIV serostatus disclosure among women in developing countries: Implications for prevention of mother-to-child transmission programmes." *Bulletin of the World Health Organization*, 82(4).

Morrell, R and Richter, L (eds). (2006) *Baba: Men and fatherhood in South Africa*. Cape Town: HSRC Press.

Nöstlinger, C; Bartoli, G; Gordillo, M; Roberfroid, D; and Colebunders, R. (2006) "Children and adolescents living with HIV positive parents: Emotional and behavioural problems." *Vulnerable Children and Youth Studies*, 1(1), 1–15.

Paiva, V; Filipe, E; Santos, N; Lima, T; and Segurado, A. (2003) "The right to love: Desire for parenthood among men living with HIV." *Reproductive Health Matters*, 11(22), 91–100.

Ramphele, M and Richter, L. (2006) "Migrancy, family dissolution and fatherhood." In Morrell, R and Richter, L (eds). *Baba: Men and fatherhood in South Africa*. Cape Town: HSRC Press.

Sherr, L and Barry, N. (2004) "Fatherhood and HIV-positive heterosexual men." *HIV Medicine*, 5(4), 258–263.

Theuring, S; Nchimbi, P; Jordan-Harder, B; and Harms, G. (2010) "Partner involvement in perinatal care and PMTCT services in Mbeya Region, Tanzania: The providers' perspective." *AIDS Care*, 22(12).

Tijou Traoré, A; Querre, M; Brou, H; Leroy, V; Desclaux, A; Desgrées-du-Loû, A. (2009) "Couples, PMTCT programs and infant feeding decision-making in Ivory Coast." *Social Science & Medicine*, 69(6), 830–837.

Daddies in the dark

Lungi Langa

Programmes that deal with the prevention of mother-to-child transmission (PMTCT) of HIV usually do not involve men. This exclusion means that mothers-to-be can withhold their positive status from their partners with relative ease. It also means that men are usually unaware that even though the mother is positive, the baby will most likely be HIV negative.

Women are often the first in a relationship to discover that they are HIV positive. Usually, this is because they are facing another consequence of having unprotected sex – pregnancy.

An expectant mother's first visit to an antenatal clinic typically involves taking an HIV test. If positive, she is immediately enrolled in a PMTCT programme. Yet many women choose not to share the process with their partners. Instead, they keep quiet, often for fear of being rejected after disclosing their status. This secrecy makes the pregnancy much harder on the woman. But it also means that the male partner remains oblivious of the threat HIV is posing to his health and the health of his future children.

Eliot and Thoko

At 32, and on the brink of fatherhood, Eliot was in the dark. He had no idea that his expectant wife, Thoko, was HIV positive. Early into her pregnancy, she left their home in Cape Town and went to stay with her family in the Eastern Cape.

While she was away, Eliot's health began to deteriorate. "I got really sick and decided to go to Site B Clinic in Khayelitsha where I was asked to give sputum for a tuberculosis test," he remembers.

The results came back positive and Eliot was immediately started on treatment.

When he remained ill even after completing the treatment, his wife's sister encouraged him to test for HIV. The result was positive. The virus had already broken down the defences of his immune system and with a CD4 count of 50, Eliot had AIDS.

"They asked me to bring my wife along, but she wasn't back yet." Eliot would later learn that Thoko had disclosed her status to her sister. "I think that is why she advised me to get tested."

When Thoko returned from the Eastern Cape, Eliot needed answers. "She told me she was tested when she found out she was pregnant. She said they put her on antiretroviral treatment," he recalls.

Early into her pregnancy, Thoko started the PMTCT programme but chose not to include Eliot. From then on, not quite knowing why, Eliot struggled to be involved in his wife's pregnancy. Every time he eagerly accompanied Thoko to the Site B Clinic, he was told to wait outside the consultation rooms for her to finish. "We [men] were not allowed to come into the antenatal meetings where the mothers waited to consult with healthcare workers," he said.

"When I asked how I would know what to do when my wife needed help or how I could keep track of the pregnancy, I was told to ask my wife. They said since she received all the information at the clinic, she should be the one who transfers it to me."

Despite his eagerness to be involved, Eliot missed most of the process. "I was not there during my daughter's birth. I only came over to pick them up the following day."

Even after his daughter was born, Eliot remained clueless. "I didn't understand why my wife insisted on not breastfeeding. I asked her, and she told me that that was the choice she made at the clinic." In reality, Thoko would have decided not to breastfeed after consultation with a healthcare practitioner. At the time, mothers were given the option to either breastfeed or formula feed exclusively.[47]

Even though it put her husband's health at risk, Thoko's failure to disclose is more likely to have been a case of fear than malicious intent. "She said she was scared that my family would think she infected me and that they would reject her," said Eliot. Fortunately for Thoko, Eliot understands his wife's dilemma. "I am just sad that many women keep their status from their partners like she did."

Since Eliot confronted Thoko, both parents are involved in their child's health. When the new baby girl was due for her first follow-up, both Eliot and Thoko were there.

But the effects of not fully involving the father still linger. "I was surprised that the baby was born HIV negative. Her being infected was one of the things I really worried about."

Where implemented correctly, babies have a less than 2 per cent chance of contracting HIV from their mothers. Knowing this could have spared Eliot a great deal of anguish. But Eliot says he is just grateful. "The most important thing for me is that my daughter was born HIV negative."

47   National guidelines on breastfeeding were changed in 2011.

Sabelo

When Sabelo Mpondo (35) discovered he was HIV positive in 2007, his wife had already died of an AIDS-related illness. Yet the 11-month-old son she left behind was HIV negative.

It was only when he started putting the pieces together that Sabelo realised his wife knew she was positive during her pregnancy. She also went through the PMTCT process without informing him. "I know she took treatment when she was pregnant. She told me it was to prevent our baby from 'being infected'. But she never told me what this infection was," he recalls.

Before their son's first birthday, Sabelo's wife died of pneumonia. Soon after, his own health began to deteriorate. It was then that he was diagnosed with HIV.

Sabelo was not very involved in his wife's pregnancy. He was working as a carpenter at the time and could not take leave to accompany his wife on her scheduled visits to the clinic.

When he was turned away from the clinic on the day his wife went into labour, he did not make much of it. "It is a common cultural belief that men should not be present during the birth of a child. Some men send their wives to stay with their mothers. The wife would leave her home pregnant and return with a baby in her arms," he says. "So I went home and planned to return to pick them both up the next day."

Spectator dads

Sabelo's case of being a father from the sidelines is not uncommon. Yet for Sabelo it meant not discovering his own HIV-positive status until much later, which had serious repercussions. "The hardest part about finding out that I was HIV positive was that I was all alone. I didn't even have a job. I was fired because I was too sick and started missing work."

The strong focus on maternal health in most PMTCT programmes means that men are frequently excluded and soon-to-be mothers are not normally encouraged to share the experience with their part-ners. Yet involving men could have a number of positive outcomes, including better adherence for the mother as well as easier imple-mentation of exclusive infant feeding. While neglecting to address men's roles as fathers has serious repercussions for the success of the PMTCT programme, it also means that an unnecessarily large number of men slip through the cracks without being admitted to an ART programme.

Names have been changed.

Fathering hope

Lungi Langa

Whether or not to have a child is often a challenging decision to make, but it is even more difficult for couples in which either one or both partners are living with HIV. Having a baby usually means having unprotected sex, but with HIV this might put your partner, or your baby, at risk.

While testing HIV positive can mean many things (including an end to some relationships), it does not have to mean the end of the dream of fatherhood. "Despite all the concerns a couple might have about HIV transmission, it is still possible to fall pregnant safely with cautious planning," says Dr Paul le Roux, a reproductive specialist at the Cape Fertility Clinic in Cape Town,

Le Roux agrees that the choice to conceive is often difficult; this is especially so in HIV serodiscordant couples (where only one partner is positive) where condoms are usually used to protect the negative partner.

While a lot of attention has been paid to preventing HIV transmission from positive mothers to their unborn babies, not enough has been said about safely conceiving in a serodiscordant partnership. In the case of an HIV-positive female and her negative partner, the risk of transmitting the virus can be relatively easily avoided by means of artificial insemination. This can be done at home at a low cost using a syringe to insert semen into the vagina. But where the male is positive, managing the risk of transmission is considerably more complex – though by no means impossible.

Two HIV-positive men from Khayelitsha shared their efforts to safely conceive HIV-negative children with their partners.

Andile

Being diagnosed with HIV in 2004 changed Andile Madondile's life drastically.

Andile (30) was ill with various symptoms, including diarrhoea and persistent headaches, forcing him to seek medical assistance. A nurse at the Site B Clinic in Khayelitsha suggested an HIV test, and the result came back positive.

"It was hard for me to accept my status. I kept it to myself for the whole week after finding out. I eventually called my mother and told her. Two weeks after finding out, I told my partner and she left me," he recalls.

Andile was left to look after their three-year-old daughter alone. He also lost his job after disclosing his status. This left him feeling "hopeless and useless". With a rope in his hand, desperate to end his misery, suicide seemed the only option.

"My daughter was outside when I decided to hang myself. But she came in and saw me hanging from the roof. She called the neighbours and they cut me down."

Thus began his road to recovery.

The first step was antiretroviral treatment. With a CD4 count of a mere 9, his immune system was severely compromised.

"Although there were side effects, I found that I was getting a lot better after starting treatment."

When Andile's ex saw his health was improving, she returned home. "She left me out of fear because she saw that I was too sick and thought I would die," he said.

Andile forgave her and in 2007 they were married. They soon started talking about starting a family. But doing that safely without infecting his partner or their baby seemed nearly impossible.

"Our only option at the time was sperm-washing, followed by

artificial insemination, which was very expensive," Andile recalls.

As HIV resides mainly in semen and not the sperm, sperm-washing can isolate the sperm by separating it from the HIV-infected seminal fluid. The "clean" sperm is then inserted into the female partner as a means of artificial insemination.

"But not before we conduct a very sensitive HIV-PCR test on the washed sperm sample to check that it is HIV negative first," explains Dr Le Roux.

Fortunately, Andile and his wife received a generous donation to undergo the procedure. Nine months later, Andile's partner – who has remained negative – gave birth to a healthy HIV-negative son.

Gcobani

Gcobani Ndumndum (29) has known he was HIV positive since he was 19. He took an HIV test in preparation for initiation camp to be circumcised. The result turned his life upside down.

"I was traumatised because I was so young. Fortunately, my family supported me and told me that I could still live even though I was HIV positive," he recalls.

In spite of his family's encouragement to treat his illness like any other chronic condition, it took Gcobani a long time before he could accept it. Unlike Andile, he kept his status hidden from his partner. He told himself he was protecting his relationship.

"From the time we started our relationship, I told her that we needed to use condoms because I had heard about HIV. Actually, I was scared to tell her. But I knew I had to eventually." That time came three years later when his partner told him that she was ready to have a baby. Gcobani had to come clean.

He immediately started researching his options. "I wanted to have a child but did not want to take the risk of infecting her," he said.

Gcobani took solace in the fact that he was not alone. "Many men like me want to have children but are afraid because of their HIV status. I went all-out to see what options were available for us. I wanted to put these to the test and see if they could work for us."

After consulting with a private practitioner, the couple opted for in vitro fertilisation (IVF), which entails extracting the eggs and fertilising them with the sperm in the laboratory. "The fertilised eggs, called embryos, are then transferred a few days later into the womb of the female partner," explains Dr Le Roux.

The procedure was successful and the couple gave birth to an HIV-negative son. Their relationship, however, did not last.

A few years later Gcobani was at a similar crossroads. He found a new partner and had to disclose – again. But this time, he says, it was easier. She was also positive and more willing to accept his status. As their relationship progressed, they decided to try for a child.

"We agreed that we would conceive by having unprotected sex. But we knew this meant effective consultations with medical practitioners because we wanted to protect our own health and ensure that our baby was not infected."

By enrolling in the PMTCT programme at their nearest clinic, the couple would be able to keep the risk of their baby contracting HIV to a minimum during the pregnancy, labour and breastfeeding. But they also needed to manage the risk of reinfecting each other during conception.

Because the HI-virus is continually mutating, there are many different types in circulation and it is possible to contract another kind of HIV even when you are already infected. This is known as superinfection and can complicate treatment. By ensuring that both their immune systems were healthy and the concentration of the virus in their blood was very low, the couple were able to minimise their risk. This meant that their CD4 counts needed to be above 400 and their viral loads virtually undetectable.

They timed their attempts to conceive with the woman's ovulation period – at least 14 days prior to her menstruation – to increase the odds of fertilisation. The couple were also discouraged from engaging in rough or violent intercourse, which could increase chances of infection.

Being involved in the process from the start allowed Gcobani the opportunity to be involved in protecting his child and his partner.

Antiretroviral treatment (ART) is making safe conception for HIV-positive men increasingly accessible. Though options such as sperm-washing and in vitro insemination may be the first choice for those accessing health care in the private sector, it often makes conception for positive men seem prohibitively expensive.

However, as in the case of Gcobani's second child, lowering the man's viral load and ensuring a healthy CD4 count is a viable, much more affordable alternative. What is critically important is that the man is looking after his health, is on treatment and joins his partner in consulting medical professionals before they attempt to conceive.

Some names have been changed.

Hope dies with him

Thabisile Dlamini

*A thin line between love and hate – drawn in a daughter's jour-
ney with her HIV-positive father. This is the first of four articles
about fathers and their children in South Africa – and the effects
HIV has on families.*

It was December, a time for joy and family. But for my father it was
a time of pain.

The sangoma threw his bones and blamed my father's ill health
on his friend and colleague. He said Mike was bewitching Father so
he could take his position at work. And just like that, a friendship
was destroyed.

Father tied red wool into a hangman's noose above his bed.

"Daddy, what's that string for?" I was 20, hungry for answers.

"Mike tried to kill me, but fortunately the sangoma stopped him.
That wool is to catch his evil ways and throw them back to him. He
will die. Soon he will hang himself and he will die for trying to take
my children's father away from them."

As educated as I was, I believed my father. I believed the sangoma and I believed that Mike Nkosi, a man I had known for many
years to be funny, smart, kind and giving, was trying to kill my father.

Father burnt stuff in his bedroom. If he wasn't burning and inhal-
ing *muti*, he was boiling potions to drink or add to his bath water.
Nonetheless he got skinnier, his hair fell out and his skin became
dry. His complexion was darker than usual and he developed sores
on his genitals and in his mouth. His back was always sore and his
head sometimes hurt so much you could see the veins in his temple
vibrating.

He was always tired, wanting nothing but to sleep. He frequently complained that his tongue felt like it was burning. He said his eyes felt heavy, as though they were falling into his skull.

I felt sorry for him. Father didn't deserve the Best Dad award, but he was still my father. And no matter how much he had hurt me in the past, it hurt a hundred times more to see him in pain.

My father was a ladies' man. He had plenty of girlfriends. He liked them young too. One Friday afternoon in 2006, father travelled to KwaZulu-Natal, saying he was going to visit relatives. But we all, including Khethiwe, knew he had a girlfriend there.

Khethiwe lived with us. We'd been told that she was my father's cousin on his father's side. I found that strange because my father always said he didn't know his father's family. Yet I believed him.

Khethiwe and I had become close. She always helped with the chores and took care of my sister and brother. She was there the Friday father left, ironing and packing his clothes for him.

That weekend was great. We had so much fun. Father was always strict and wanted to keep us indoors, even though I was 20 and Khetiwe 26. Looking back, I'm certain he thought we'd witness his behaviour if we were in the streets after dark. He was the kind of 40-plus man you would bump into at a club, a twenty-first birthday or a Chomee concert.

That weekend, we celebrated our freedom before "the warden" was due back. Khethiwe and I stole father's bottle of Amarula and drank it like it was juice. We agreed that we would say the bottle fell and broke. But that Sunday, when father returned, there was so much drama, the Amarula didn't matter.

"Meet my eldest Thokozile, my second-born Thembakazi and the last-born Sibusiso," said my father. "Next to me is my cousin from my dad's side of the family."

Father had arrived home with a chubby woman in a bright orange, traditional Xhosa garment. There was a slight pause and then we greeted her.

My father sighed, then added: "Right, this is Khanyi and she is … *uhm* … she is the woman I want to spend the rest of my life with … I trust we will make her feel welcome."

Nobody said a word and father told Khanyi to follow him to the bedroom. Khethiwe broke into tears.

"He should marry me," she said. "He forced me to have two abortions." My suspicions were finally confirmed. Khethiwe and my father were lovers.

Father had lied to his family and, truth be told, he didn't love that poor girl. She was there, she was naïve and he couldn't keep his pants on. They had cooked up the cousin story because Khethiwe did indeed have the same surname as my dad's father. It was just a coincidence.

My father had done some bad things in his life but this was unforgivable. I felt like an outsider in my own home. I felt that my father didn't give a damn how I felt about anything.

My half-siblings were still very young. Sibusiso was only six years old. All he did was play, eat and sleep. But Thembakazi was 11 and she got along with Khanyi just fine. After her mom had died in 2004, she had longed to have a mom. I was 21 by now and I handled the situation by staying out of her way. I never gave her reason to say anything to me. If we didn't speak and I was seldom home, then we wouldn't fight.

A few months later Khanyi was pregnant. And my father was unemployed and terribly ill. One day, rummaging through Khanyi's personal belongings, I found her clinic card. Truth is, I was snooping for a reason to hate my father even more – and I found one. It was a birth date: 17 August 1987. Khanyi was only three days older than me.

The day Khanyi gave birth she didn't have any clothes for the child and few for herself. Father gave her my brand-new jersey to wear to the hospital.

The baby girl had jaundice and stayed in the hospital for a week. I was working part-time and studying. My fees were in arrears and I was locked out from school on many occasions. The money I earned was not enough to get myself through college. But when I was paid that month, I spent my entire earnings on the baby's clothes, napkins, wipes and milk.

Father was happy and thanked me over and over. Then he made what appeared to be a random comment: "Khanyi got tested for HIV, you know, and she's clean. So I know I'm fine. It's Mike and his *muti* that he's using to bewitch me."

The baby died three months later. Khanyi returned to KwaZulu-Natal, leaving my father desperately ill. I feared he would take his last breath at any moment. Khethiwe was nowhere to be found.

Father had consulted a number of general practitioners, but each on a single complaint: a headache or a stomach pain. Each had prescribed for that condition, but he never got better. He also started forgetting things. Sometimes he wouldn't recognise family members and neighbours. I told him he needed to get tested for HIV. He kept telling me that Khanyi had tested negative, which meant he was fine. I persisted though.

A part of me wanted him to be HIV positive because then we'd know what was wrong. If the test came back positive, we'd get him treatment. If the test came back negative, we were back to square one – not knowing what to do.

Going for the test was a nightmare. The taxi driver demanded the passengers board four-four on the seats. Father was terribly uncomfortable, saying his body was in unbearable pain.

From the taxi stop, we had to walk almost a kilometre. It felt like five. Every few steps, father had to sit down on the pavement. Every time he sat down, I was afraid he wouldn't be able to get up again.

At the testing station, father went in alone. I skimmed through magazines and HIV pamphlets and allowed my mind to drift. I imagined my father recovered and healthy again. A movie was playing in my mind. In the first scene, a psychologist helped us forget the past, fix the present and be happy in the future. Father asked for forgiveness and told me something I had never heard come out of his mouth: "I love you." We hugged and …

"Thokozile, come!" I was following him when he stopped, lifted his arms and dropped them again,

"They say I've got it." Then he continued walking.

To my surprise he didn't seem shocked. On the way home, all I could think of was the dishonesty. Either Khanyi had lied to my father or Father had lied to me. Then again, maybe he had lied to himself.

Less than a week later, we discovered that father's CD4 count was at a low 23. The virus was widespread in his body. He had AIDS.

He fought with the nurse trying to take his blood. "I'm clean," he shouted. "You're trying to infect me with HIV." I was desperate for him to get help and it took all my determination to calm him down. I wanted my father to be healthy again. I needed him to take care of his kids. I wasn't ready to carry the responsibility of a 7-year-old boy and a 12-year-old girl.

The nurse said it was going to take about two weeks to get his antiretrovirals. In my mind he didn't have two weeks. I begged her to help him live. She went to the back and came out with a brown paper bag.

"What I'm doing is not allowed. I could get into a lot of trouble … I hope that by the time this patient is due to pick up his ARVs, your father's order is ready."

She begged me to make sure he didn't default. She told my father the side effects might be severe but that, after a while, they would go away. Father promised he would take the medication. I gave him a hug and told him I would be there for him. I didn't ask what we were going to do.

The nurse told my father he was lucky. "Your daughter loves you, Mr Sibiya. She wants you to survive and, if you work together, you'll recover. I've seen miracles."

He didn't keep his promise.

Once I caught him taking the pills out of his mouth when he thought I wasn't looking. So after he took his ARVs, I had to make him open his mouth and move his tongue around. He said that, because I was educated, I believed in white people's explanations. He said he was an African man and that he was going to heal himself the African way.

"I'm not taking these stupid pills any more. I don't want them. Do you hear me? I don't want them!"

"You're going to die," I wanted to say.

I told him the sangoma wasn't going to help. "You know nothing about your culture and your roots," he told me.

He stopped trusting me. When I cooked, he wouldn't eat until I had tasted the food first. He said I was trying to poison him.

They say the eyes are the windows to the soul. Looking into my father's eyes, I tried to find him buried in all the pain, all the confusion and all the fear. But he was gone. He was still breathing, but he was no longer there.

It was hard to survive. The money I earned went on transport to the kids' school and my work. I used the rest to buy food, but it didn't last the month.

Father had another house, which he put on the market. I was relieved. When the money came in, he said he would give me R5000 to spoil myself. But he was happy with me one day, cracking jokes and laughing, and would shut me out the next.

When the money was transferred, I reminded him about my school fees, but all he said was: "I don't care." Later, I discovered he had given Khethiwe R3000 to register for a computer course.

Father had money and he felt invincible. As ill as he was, he bought a new car. Thembakazi told me his hand was too weak to change gears. He was coaching her to change them for him.

On the road at night, he would sometimes pull over to sleep. I told the kids not to travel with him but they loved him – and they loved that new car. He took them to McDonald's, bought them clothes and gave them money. All I could do was pray for their safety.

Father wasn't safe at all. My uncle told him to visit a traditional healer. He said HIV was a white man's way of killing black people. He brought herbs and they boiled their potion on the stove. It smelt terrible. Father drank it and my uncle assured him he would be healed in no time.

Out of the blue, he developed a hatred for Thembakazi. It was December. A time for the old township tradition: kids showing off their new clothes on Christmas Day. Father had bought Sibusiso new clothes and shoes. Thembakazi got nothing.

"You've formed an alliance with your sister so ask her for money to buy clothes." She wept for hours.

Father and Sibusiso now travelled alone. Father said he didn't want to be separated from his son. The little girl was distraught.

By this stage Khethiwe was back in the picture and I had had enough. I had headaches and fatigue. My shoulders were stiff and my back sore. The doctor diagnosed stress and depression. She said I would have a heart attack if I carried on that way.

To escape, I moved in with my boyfriend. I had to get away from Father, for my own health. I would be of no use to the children if I were ill. But every day, I prayed that God would protect them.

It was a Monday morning. I don't think he knew I was there. His eyes were closed and he was breathing heavily. He had foam in his mouth.

He was helpless. It was unbelievable. The soldier had fallen on his sword, but somehow the sword had pierced my heart. He was no longer able to shout at me, insult me, beat me or lie to me. Yet, at that moment, I would have given anything for him to wake up and cause me all that pain again.

He had been an abusive man. Yet I wanted to experience the abuse again because at least the abuser would be alive. I loved him. I wasn't ready to let go.

I skipped Tuesday and decided I would see him again on Wednesday. The hospital called to say he died on Tuesday night.

The hope of things improving between us died with him. The chance of a better relationship disappeared.

At that moment, I hated him all over again.

Names have been changed.

"My daughter kept me going"
Thabisile Dlamini

Lerato didn't remember her father. When he returned after eight years, he carried regret, love ... and HIV. This is the second in a series of four articles about fathers and their children in South Africa – and the effects HIV has on families.

When Lerato was 12, she arrived home from school to find two men sitting with her mother. She didn't recognise either of them.

After a few minutes studying their faces, one of the men started to look familiar, but she couldn't remember where she had seen him. Lerato ran to her bedroom and began looking through old pictures. And there he was. In one of Lerato's baby pictures, he was holding her to face the camera. The man in the other room was her father.

Not knowing your own father is a reality for millions of children in South Africa. The Human Sciences Research Council (HSRC) reports that 57 per cent of all children and 63 per cent of African children have fathers who are either absent or dead.

The last time Mduduzi saw Lerato she was four years old. Eight years later, she came face to face with the man she had wanted to confront ever since she was old enough to realise that other kids had fathers and she didn't.

All it would take was one sentence: Why did you leave me? But the words choked her and, instead of spitting them out, she swallowed.

"It wasn't how I had pictured meeting my dad."

Lerato had envisioned this particular scene many times. It was an important scene in the movie of her life. The reel lay in the back of her head, stored for the day it would really happen. In the movie, Lerato was prepared. Mduduzi didn't come unannounced.

He knocked on the door. He sat down and introduced himself. He explained why he hadn't been around. And he had a good reason. The reel never quite ran to the point where she heard his reason. But she knew it would make sense … unlike the reason she heard in real life.

"Your grandmother made your mother choose between me, the father of her baby, and her. I was unemployed and unable to look after both you and your mother. She was still in high school and chose to stay with her mother, who could care for the both of you."

Mduduzi still says he had no choice, but Lerato thinks that's just an excuse. Many unanswered questions linger in the girl's mind. But asking them now might open old wounds. So, mostly, she decides to let them go.

The girl who met her father at 12 is now 15. They're having lunch together in Soweto. Mduduzi is bragging that his daughter is a clever child at school. But Lerato interrupts: "I'm in Grade 10 now. I know you don't know. And by the way, I almost failed Grade 8."

"Failed? Why?"

"Because I was 13 and there was so much going on in my life."

Tears flood her brown eyes. She blinks repeatedly. "I had to see a counsellor recommended by the school," she says. "My father doesn't even know that."

Mduduzi looks away, staring out the window as the girl recalls why she will never forget age 13.

"I knew there was something wrong with my father – but I didn't think it was this serious."

Mduduzi was keeping a secret from his daughter. But somehow he just couldn't find the words to tell her. Sometimes he thought he had them. Sentences would construct themselves in his head, ready to make their way out of his mouth. But looking his daughter straight in the face, his heart would beat faster and he'd start shaking.

"Daddy, are you okay? Should I call for help?" she asked him.

"No, just bring me a glass of water."

He couldn't do it. He couldn't tell her. But somehow, she had to know.

Lerato recalls the meeting as if it were an exam she had to pass. It was between herself, her father and a social worker. Less than a year before, her father had walked back into her life. She was only just starting to forgive him; to open up and trust him again.

"Your father is HIV positive," the social worker told her. Her father remained silent.

"Is he going to die?"

Lerato took a while to process the information. They had been taught about HIV at school, but she had never imagined that some-one in her family could have it. Especially not her long-lost father, who had arrived back in her life to save her from a completely father-less childhood.

The girl was distraught. After so many years, growing up without her father, he was back. And now he was HIV positive.

"I was shocked. He was back to be my hero. I wasn't expecting my hero to be sick."

As she remembers that day, Lerato's eyes finally spill over. "My father once said, when he is sick he wants me around because I make him feel better."

Mduduzi nods. "It's true. Sometimes I feel very weak and I start thinking about my daughter. She is my only child and yet I've wasted so much time depriving us of each other. When my daughter is near I feel strong."

Before Mduduzi came back into his daughter's life, he was admitted to Chris Hani Baragwanath Hospital in Soweto, having suffered a stroke. He remained under medical care for two months. From his hospital room window, he had a bird's-eye view of Diepkloof Zone 3. That was where his child was.

"My daughter kept me going. I was determined to be healthy again so we could be together."

The 35-year-old father was diagnosed with HIV in the year 2000. "I'm still going to live a long life. I might not live to see my sixties but I am not dying soon. I have a daughter to live for."

Lerato smiles, drawing an answering smile from her father. Then he bursts into laughter.

"Don't mind me. I'm just thinking. Lerato acts like a nurse sometimes. It's funny."

"I don't act like a nurse!"

"Oh really?" Mduduzi places his hands on his hips and, speaks in falsetto: "Where are you going? When are you coming back? Don't forget those things!" The things being Mduduzi's antiretrovirals.

"She won't allow me to carry her schoolbag." Role-playing again, Mduduzi pouts: "It's too heavy for you, I'll manage!"

Lerato teases him back. "Let me see your cellphone. It's so outdated. Daddy, it's a kiddie's phone." He laughs.

Drinking from the same litre-bottle of Coke, father and daughter argue about a family wedding Mduduzi had invited Lerato to. "You told me there was a wedding. You didn't say when and where it was going to be. And I've told you a million times before that, if you want me to visit, you must phone my mother."

"Why should I ask her for permission for my own child to visit me?"

"Because she raised me and she has legal custody," Lerato tells him firmly. The discussion heats up and Lerato admits to breaking a promise she made to her father. "I told my mother about your status."

Mduduzi is speechless for a moment. Then he says: "I can see the smirk on her face already. 'Yah, he's got AIDS!' Why did you tell her after I asked you not to?" Shaking his head he puts his food down and sips on the Coke.

"Do you love me?" Lerato asks in reply.

"Of course I love you."

"I know you do. I just wonder sometimes if you want to have a proper relationship with me. Things are okay, but they can be better … I don't just want to see you now, and then see you again three months later. I want us to have a proper relationship where we see each other often."

Mduduzi says he wants that too but … "If I had a job I would go to Diepkloof and do the right thing according to our culture. I would pay your family what I owe them, buy myself a house and have you live with me. But I'm unemployed, I still live in my parents' house and I sometimes feel …"

"Feel what?"

"It's hard to explain. If I had a job, our relationship would be better, but things are not going well for me."

"That's the problem with my dad," Lerato comments. "He doesn't understand that money is not going to make me happy. I'm already scared we don't have enough time. All I want is to see him regularly and be able to call him anytime I need to talk. I want him to understand me and make the effort to be involved in my life."

Sipping their Coke, father and daughter begin to talk about how they could strengthen their relationship. They conclude that they need to do things together. Things that don't involve money. Things like taking a walk in the park, doing school assignments and cooking.

"And watching TV," Mduduzi adds.

"Watching TV? Wow, I have a cool dad."

"Programmes like *Soul City*. You're in a very dangerous stage of your life right now and it's time to get all the information you need to protect yourself from HIV. Trust me, you don't want this disease."

Instead of answering, Lerato grabs the bottle of Coke and drinks from it.

"Concentrate on school," he adds. "It will keep you out of trouble."

"I will. I love school. Call my mom. I want to visit during the school holidays."

Names have been changed.

Pride and paternity

Thabisile Dlamini

Mandla believes he disappointed his father. Yet he doesn't see his own child because he can't provide for him financially. This is the third in a series of four articles about fathers and their children in South Africa – and the effects HIV has on families.

Mandla Ngobese says he has a close relationship with his son.

"How old is he?"

"About 11 or 12."

"Which school does he attend?"

"Eish! I forgot the name of his school."

"What grade is he in?"

"Uhm, what grade are 11-year-olds usually in?"

"How often do you see him?" Mandla scratches his head, but doesn't answer.

The mother of Mandla's son died in 2007 from AIDS-related illnesses. The little boy now lives with his grandmother – one of 63 per cent of African children in South Africa who don't live with their fathers. Some of those fathers have died. Others, like Mandla, are simply absent.

Mandla was infected with HIV in 1997, but disclosed his status to his family in 1999. In 2003 he had a stroke and began antiretroviral treatment two years later.

"I am very open with my child," says the 38-year-old father, but later says he isn't sure if his son is aware of his HIV status. "I didn't tell him, but the family knows, so he must have overheard them speaking about it."

Mandla still carries evidence of the stroke in his gait. His hands shake as he struggles to hold a coffee mug in one hand, and twists the tap open with the other. Limping to his seat, Mandla pulls an album from his wardrobe and pages through family photographs.

His own mother died when he was eight. He was raised by his father. Mandla had the chance to form a relationship with his own father, yet he believes he disappointed him. He says he didn't deserve the love he got from him.

"My father was not educated, especially not about HIV. But he was a traditional African man and he believed that he was steering me in the right direction. He loved me. He wanted to help me."

His father died last year at the age of 61. "He was ill for a very long time and, because he didn't believe in Western medicine, we never found out what was wrong with him."

Before his stroke, Mandla was able to work. "Life was good back then. Now I don't have money. I rely on the grant and they will cut it when my CD4 count rises. That is why I hardly see my child. His mother's family thinks I am useless because I cannot afford to take care of him. They told my son that I was not worthy to be called a dad. I am very lucky that my father left me this house or else I would be homeless."

Phyllis Maseko, a social worker in the Ekurhuleni district, believes unemployment often causes fathers to feel they are not "man enough" to support their children financially. "Hence the shame makes them stay away from their children."

Before his father died, Mandla's relationship with him was also characterised by shame. After he was diagnosed with HIV, he didn't feel worthy to be his father's son.

His father told him it was "a white man's disease". He said Mandla didn't have HIV, he had *umuhlwa* – a disease believed to be caused by sleeping with a woman who had an abortion and failed to have a traditional cleansing ceremony. In the township, sleeping with a woman who has had an abortion is considered a disgrace – and a health risk if she has not had a cleansing ceremony.

"I hated my father thinking that of me. It was humiliating."

Father and son moved from one sangoma to the next, hoping Mandla would be healed. But his health kept fluctuating. He was fine one week, feeble the next. Mandla was 28 at the time. His father was 52. It was 1999 and talking about HIV was taboo.

"People did not have enough knowledge about the virus. I know I didn't. This was the same era when plenty of people in the black culture believed that white people were injecting HIV-infected blood into oranges to kill the black nation."

The oranges were red inside – because they were not oranges. They were grapefruit. Mandla knows that now. But he didn't back in 1999, when all he could do was speculate. And his father, a traditional man, drummed into him that "HIV does not exist".

"There were no HIV support groups at the time and the information was not readily available. Because of ignorance, I must have infected about five women after knowing about my status – one of them being the mother of my son."

Phyllis, who works with many families in the same situation, believes Mandla could turn things around with his own son. "He is in a better position to teach and get through to his child by making an example of himself. His child could learn a lot from him ... All children need and want fathers. Young men, especially, need older male role models or father figures to guide them on life skills, advising them against crime and risky sexual behaviour."

Fathers who think their only responsibility is financial are not looking at the bigger picture. "There are plenty of ways to prove your love for your children other than money," says Phyllis. "You can spend time with them, play with them, help them with their homework, hug them and tell them you love them ... The simplest meal served with love is better than a gourmet dish with a sore heart yearning for a neglectful father to change."

Phyllis says children have deep internal scars from the absence of their fathers. "They feel as though they are not loved."

Professor Linda Richter, executive director of Child, Youth and Family Development, agrees. "In a country where fathers are absent from homes and the lives of their children, they still feature strongly in the minds and yearnings of young people, including young men at risk of contracting HIV."

Mandla is on ARVs and no longer relies on traditional healers. Yet he still believes his stroke was caused by witchcraft.

"I was working at the Vodacom public phones. One day, I was at work and I just collapsed. When I was working I was able to send money for my son. They bewitched me because of jealousy. Whoever did this to me was jealous that I was taking care of my son.

"I'll never find a job. Who would hire me? Look at me. I'm just living day by day. Life doesn't make sense."

One thing does still give Mandla pride. He stands and pulls a drawer open. It's time to take his ARVs. Despite the side effects when he began taking them, he never gave up.

"Since 2005 I've never stopped taking these. I've never relapsed."

Names have been changed.

The all-around father

Thabisile Dlamini

"Daddy has to work so he has another family that he lives with closer to his job!" This is the last in a series of four articles about fathers and their children in South Africa – and the effects HIV has on families.

Nhlanhla Mavundla's youngest child is four months old. The 35-year-old AIDS activist was present at the birth and says the event is tattooed on his mind. "She is very beautiful."

He speaks equally proudly of his other children. "My oldest son is 11, my daughter is nine … and I have another little girl."

"How old is your little girl?"

Nhlanhla changes the subject. Later, the conversation returns to children and the question is raised again. "How old is your little girl?"

Nhlanhla pauses. "Seven months."

"Seven months … but your youngest is four months."

Nhlanhla looks away, fixing his eyes on the bird building a nest in a nearby tree. Pointing, he says, "I provide for my children. They have food, clothes and a roof over their heads."

Nhlanhla manages several HIV and AIDS support groups in Soweto under a very large organisation. He does school visits and speaks to young people about HIV, always disclosing his status. His position makes him a role model for his community.

"In the beginning I was afraid that I was going to die and my children would grow up without a father. But I've been on antiretroviral treatment for two years now and my CD4 count is very high."

Nhlanhla has known that he was HIV positive for nine years now, but nonetheless admits to having unprotected sex with different women. The evidence would be hard to deny.

"I used to live in Thembisa with the mother of my three children. We separated for a little while. During our separation I met someone else. By the time I found out she was pregnant, so was the woman I was living with in Soweto ... Even on the day she was giving birth she didn't tell me. I found out from my aunt that she was in labour at the hospital."

Nhlanhla, dark-skinned and handsome, with a gold tooth, is "still together" with the mother of his three children, but also lives with the other woman. He is not married to either of them.

"It does trouble me sometimes. The children know they have a sister in Soweto, but it's always hard to juggle, giving the same attention to all my children."

As an AIDS activist, Nhlanhla has all the information he needs to protect himself – and the women he is intimate with. Inevitably, the conversation touches on his concerns. Is he worried about infecting the women he sleeps with or being reinfected himself?

"I am open about my status. I don't hide it from them."

Nhlanhla will say no more than that. He remains silent, and then adds: "Both the mothers of my children are HIV positive, but all my children are HIV negative. The mothers were on AZT." Nhanhla speaks confidently, sure of his facts.

Nhlanhla admits that he sleeps around. "I am a man," he says.

And yet he believes the mother of his first three children infected him. "The first mother of my children found out her HIV status before me. She was cheating on me. But I'm over it."

It is a Saturday. Nhlanhla is to speak at an AIDS awareness event at the Snaoane Community Hall & Swimming Pool in Soweto. Eleven-year-old Siphiwe and nine-year-old Nomfundo sit side by side, watching their father speak of prevention and ARVs, disclosing his own status as he does so.

"My father is teaching people about HIV, so they don't get sick," says the boy. Siphiwe says he knows about HIV. He knows that "if you don't take your medicine, you will get very sick".

"I have two little sisters," says Nomfundo with a big smile carved out of ice cream. And yes, she says, they are a family. Dad lives with another woman, but comes to see them often – and sleeps in Mommy's bedroom.

"My daddy has to work in Soweto so he lives with Aunt Karabo but he comes to see us in Thembisa and sometimes stays for the weekend with my mother."

"When my daddy comes he brings nice food and sometimes clothes," adds Siphiwe, who is clothed in Nike from top to toe.

"He also takes us to KFC," Nomfundo murmurs, licking at her fast-collapsing ice cream.

Nhlanhla says his children are fine. They are doing well, and he believes he is doing his best to be a good father to them. "I take care of them. That is what a father is supposed to do, isn't it?"

Nhlanhla's situation is not uncommon. Social worker Phyillis Maseko is not surprised. She works with many families and has seen it all before. She has her own opinions, though, of the children's easy acceptance: "When children are that young, they forgive easily. But then they grow up, they start analysing things more closely – things they may not be able to come right out and talk about. Then they become bitter."

Phyllis believes Nhlanhla's children will start to ask questions as they grow older. "Their father comes to see them bearing gifts and they look forward to his visits. But because he is not there 24/7, and they know he is with another family, chances are they will feel cheated and want more."

The situation holds potential for a lot more complications, particularly while Nhlanhla refuses to choose between them. "It's confusing for the children. They won't admit it to their parents but, trust me, they are not really comfortable with the situation."

Names have been changed.

Men who have sex with men

"I was pissed off with myself. We weren't laaities *any more and should have been able to control our urges. But I thought what my wife and kids didn't know wouldn't hurt them."*

"On Saturdays I'm gay and do boys. On Sundays I'm playing straight and go for girls."

Men who have sex with men / Introduction

The journalism in this section was written by Pieter van Zyl during his fellowship with the project in 2009. Rather than rely on the very limiting and worn-out "gay" label, Van Zyl's coverage sketches nuanced portraits of complex and diverse men, offering a perspective on alternative male sexuality and experience that goes beyond the more common (and often stereotypical) images of openly gay men.

While all of these men are having sex with men, they have not always considered themselves gay, and some still do not. Thus, for Hendrik in Van Zyl's first article titled "Brokeback Marriage", it is only after decades of denial, guilt and secret gay sex that he finally opens up to his family and wife. It takes him even longer still to enter into his first openly gay relationship. Many of the men who frequent Bra Mo's place looking for male sexual companions in "After nine at Bra Mo's", on the other hand, flat-out reject the label "gay".

Though the characters in Van Zyl's stories all differ vastly from each other, all of them can be broadly classed as *men who have sex with men* (MSM). Commonly misunderstood to equate to "being gay", the term MSM is used in HIV and sexual health contexts to accommodate all men who engage in same-sex activity, regardless of whether they choose to (openly) label themselves "gay" or not.

MSM have always faced higher risks of contracting HIV. Part of this can be attributed to the heightened biological risk associated with anal sex.[1] But the risk of contracting HIV is also considerably higher for MSM living in countries where stigma and prejudice are rife.[2] In sub-Saharan Africa, presidents and respected community

---

1   The probability of contracting HIV during unprotected receptive anal sex can be up to 18 times greater than during vaginal intercourse (Baggaley, White and Boily, 2010).

2   The World Health Organization (WHO) estimates that in low- and middle-income countries MSM are up to 19.3 times more likely to be HIV infected than the general population (WHO, 2011).

leaders continue to openly condemn same-sex practice and throw their weight behind narrowly defined notions of what it means to be a man. Studies have estimated that HIV prevalence could be as high as 31 per cent among MSM in an environment where the rates are around 13 per cent in the general adult male population.[3]

In Hendrik's case, it is the guilt that ensues from his struggle to balance his own desires with social expectation and the threat of stigma that drives him to take risky sexual decisions, eventually resulting in HIV infection. While Hendrik eventually "comes out", despite severe prejudice, some men who are attracted to other men will never be comfortable with the gay label. It is here that stigma and prejudice directed at MSM have the most direct impact on the HIV epidemic. Like some of the men at Bra Mo's place, these men lead double lives – one in which they have girlfriends or wives and play into the traditional notion of manhood, and another that begins after nine in the evenings, in which they live out their sexual desires and covet men. In the townships these men are known as "after nines".[4] Their sexual encounters are rushed and often laden with guilt. These pressured rendezvous leave little time for negotiating protection and appropriate safe-sex messages, and tools for prevention (condoms and water-based lubricant) rarely reach them.

By spending time in the townships on the outskirts of Cape Town, Van Zyl could acquaint himself with the cultural subtexts that inform this high-risk environment and was able to gain insight into

---

3   Lane, Fisher Raymond, Dladla, Rosethe, Struthers, McFarland and McIntyre (2011), in a study of HIV prevalence among men in Soweto, found that among gay-identified men HIV prevalence was 33.9 per cent, with overall prevalence among the group assessed (including non-gay identifying MSM) at 13.2 per cent. The Actuarial Society of South Africa (2008) places overall prevalence among males aged 15–49 at 12.8 per cent for 2012.

4   Among others, Sjolund (2011) and Badat (2007) provide descriptions of the "after nine" lifestyles.

how MSM have chosen to respond to these challenges. Stigma and associated HIV risk thus form a subtle leitmotif throughout Van Zyl's work. These stories hold clues as to how MSM's sexual health might be better addressed. Among others, it becomes apparent that truly effective HIV intervention would not only target MSM directly, but would also include their environment.[5] Ronnie, through his generous spirit, and Frik, through his art, offer two examples of how openly gay men are helping to introduce alternative masculinities to communities and, in so doing, are helping to change people's minds and ameliorate prejudice.

Through Van Zyl's coverage, it also becomes clear why behaviour-change campaigns often miss the mark when it comes to MSM. The vast majority of existing safe-sex messages tap into traditional ideas of masculinity, not only ostracising MSM but reinforcing existing traditional masculine ideals. Messages aimed at the homosexual contingent, on the other hand, tend to be too overtly gay and miss the mark for non-gay-identifying MSM. Effectively reaching this group requires subtle, low-key messaging that emphasises behaviours rather than identities.[6] The poster in Bra Mo's place is one example of a tailored message that takes into account the various complexities that inform MSM. Without offering any detail, it simply announces: "This is my house, don't judge what I'm doing." It forms part of Bra Mo's philosophy of providing men with a space to be themselves and love who they want.

Bra Mo works at a local clinic and is well aware of the HIV risks inherent in clandestine, rushed sex – though not all clinic staff share

---

5   By way of example, Health4Men has launched campaigns to this effect in townships in Cape Town and Soweto where, with a series of posters, social events and networking activities, they are seeking to change people's minds about same-sex relationships and behaviour. For more, visit Health4Men at www.health4men.co.za.

6   Jobson (2010).

his attitude. For the large part, the healthcare system is hostile and often technically ignorant to the specific needs of MSM. South African men's reported experiences of public healthcare sketch a disconcerting picture of stigma and verbal harassment.[7] A mere handful of clinic spaces cater for the specific needs of MSM and, while some effort has been made at sensitising healthcare workers and making them more "sex-positive", hostility remains extremely prevalent, putting countless men off seeking critically important sexual healthcare.[8] By covering former local soapie star Renaldo Adams's work at Health4Men, which offers a prejudice-free environment for MSM to access sexual healthcare, the journalism also highlights how desperately needed these services are.

Despite the fact that HIV remains a primary antagonist throughout Van Zyl's journalism, rather than allow it to take centre stage, he has positioned HIV as a quiet, lurking threat. It is only in the final story, as Van Zyl records the life-changing impact of acquiring the virus, where HIV is afforded a leading role. By telling the story of how one night in a police holding cell changed a gay couple's lives forever, the article highlights the all-too-common occurrence of male rape in detention. Though the experience is harrowing, detailed and accurate reporting highlights the life-saving properties of antiretroviral treatment, offering a poignant counterpoint to the couple's tragic experience.

Like the HIV rape story, all of Van Zyl's work is carefully projected against a well-researched background of stigma and high-risk behaviour. This provides continued reminders of how the social context can drive MSM further underground, increasing their likelihood

---

7   Lane, Mogale, Struthers, McIntyre and Kegeles (2008).

8   See, for instance, Health4Men's manual *From top to bottom: A sex-positive approach for men who have sex with men*, designed for healthcare practitioners, available from: http://www.anovahealth.co.za/resources/entry/toptobottom/.

of engaging in risky sexual behaviour. But while he is writing about a group of men, Van Zyl's focus at all times remains on the individuality of his characters (rather than their sexual preference). This allows them to blend with their surroundings and renders them ordinary citizens to a point where they could be anyone's brother, father, friend or neighbour. This facilitates insight that extends far beyond the scope of most coverage.

Despite the quality of the reporting and the engaging content, the mainstream print media expressed reluctance at reproducing Van Zyl's stories. A notable exception was *Drum* magazine's enthusiasm for the article detailing former soapie star Renaldo Adams's journey with HIV, probably helped along by the story's celebrity factor. Niche arts magazine *De Kat* later also picked up the story of township creative Frikkie, whose prints and paintings likely resonated with the publication's penchant for expressive art forms. The remainder of Van Zyl's journalism was published on the Health24.com platform.

Scandal and sensation: Media images of men who have sex with men

While our analysis showed the media did engage with issues around homosexuality, much of it relied on clichéd images of openly gay men – the entertainer, gay rights activist or victim of harassment. A significant proportion of the coverage often treated gay men as a faceless demographic minority – notably stories on political developments and research.[9]

Most of the coverage relied heavily on the "gay" label as men who

9 Our year-long investigation ran from March 2011 to 2012, during which only 44 articles were found featuring the keywords "gay" or "homosexual". Of those, a mere 21 mentioned HIV. Additionally, newspapers were scanned by a trained researcher to include articles that alluded to same-sex activity, even though they did not contain the keywords.

were openly sleeping with other men, featuring minimal engagement with the complexities that underwrite sexual identity, preference and behaviour. Sophisticated journalistic portrayals of MSM and mindful exploration of the stigma and prejudice that are so detrimental to the sexual health of this group were notably rare. Only seven articles (out of a total of 44) in our research attempted to paint a more nuanced picture that included prejudice and HIV and treated MSM as a diverse group of not always openly gay men.

Though coverage of MSM was thinner than anticipated, the topic does appear to have some sustained news value. This was particularly the case where gay men's issues or experiences dovetailed with matters that already had discernible news value. These included certain "hot" issues, specifically political conflict, violence, breakthroughs in science and medicine, and entertainment.

Gay men make headlines in politics and murder stories

During our period of interest, coverage was clearly dominated by battles on the political front.[10] Sadly, this was less a matter of leadership engaging in meaningful discussions around the rights of sexual minorities, and more a case of someone having put their foot in their mouth. This included Zimbabwean president Robert Mugabe's homophobic ranting, Zulu leader King Goodwill Zwelithini's assertion that gay men are "rotten" and the passing of a "guilty" verdict for South Africa's ambassador to Uganda, John Qwelane, who uttered homophobic hate speech. Some coverage was also dedicated to the voting in of a controversial so-called "anti-gay bill" in Nigeria.

---

10 During the study period, a total of 16 articles featured the key words "gay" or "homosexual" in reference to political leaders or debates. Of those political news items, four made mention of HIV.

Despite these issues relating to the perpetuation of stigma and prejudice, which has clear implications for HIV treatment and prevention, the coverage failed to make that connection. Instead, articles gave only a blow-by-blow overview of who said what. The only exception being a SAPA-AFP article published in the *Sowetan* that engages with attitudes and policy around same-sex behaviour in Botswana.[11] With a tapestry of quotes, the article manages a fairly complex description of how homophobic attitudes and legislation impact individual rights and HIV-prevention efforts at large.

This example notwithstanding, some coverage in the study was of a spate of murders for which the motive appears to have been the victims' sexual orientation. These were typical crime reports, but framed as hate crimes, possibly of a serial nature. Two of the four articles mentioned HIV, but only because one of the victims was HIV activist Jason Wessenaar.

Gay men in HIV coverage: Skimming the surface

Only 14 news articles in our analysis made clear and direct links between same-sex behaviour and HIV risk. Of these, five items could be categorised as entertainment news – two chronicled Freddie Mercury's life, marking 20 years since his death due to AIDS-related causes; a further two covered local gay celebrity Koyo Bala's disclosure of his HIV status; and the fifth promoted a series of gay stage productions. Within this group, four more articles took a biomedical or research angle – the release of new HIV prevalence figures among MSM in Soweto, a conference on the sexual health of MSM and a news short announcing the opening of an MSM-friendly clinic in Bali.

---

11   SAPA-AFP. "Sexuality debate rips Botswana apart – Is homosexuality un-African?" *Sowetan* (17 March 2011).

Of the 14 articles that engaged with HIV, only three offered context, describing how prejudice and stigma informed HIV risk. One particularly well-crafted article examines prejudice and homophobia in the public health sector and imposes this on South Africa's tense history of racism, resulting in a layered piece that leaves readers mulling over their own preconceived notions of race, sexual orientation and HIV status.[12] The other two articles are both vignettes relating to MSM services rendered by Health4Men in Cape Town, published as a set on World AIDS Day. In the first, Zack Smit, a client at the clinic, recounts his experiences being stigmatised and judged at public health facilities.[13] The other article profiles Dr Kevin Rebe from Health4Men and draws attention to the double stigma that MSM living with HIV face.[14]

The period of analysis also saw the release of the controversial Afrikaans film *Skoonheid*, which received the Queer Palm Award 2011 at Cannes. *Skoonheid* does well to highlight the difficult terrain many South African men who have sex with men must traverse. Yet, despite its acclaim and resonance, one news report speaks of the many walkouts during the film's premier.[15] The article puts this down to prejudice, or more precisely, homophobia, but does not draw parallels between the audience's repugnance at the same sex-behaviour in the film and the stigma that drove the film's characters to lead double lives. None of the coverage mentions HIV.

Though not directly part of the study findings, some of the news in the period of interest alluded to same-sex activity, yet managed to neatly circumnavigate the issue missing an opportunity to gener-

---

12   Malan, M. "Saved by 'township treatment'", *Mail & Guardian*, Health Supplement (November 2011).

13   Thom, A. "Clinic gave me second chance, says sex-addict", *The Star* (December 2011).

14   Thom, A. "Fighting a double stigma", *The Star* (December 2011).

15   Nicholson, Z. "Gay film walkouts no surprise", *The Star* (August 2011).

ate much-needed awareness among readers. Notably, this included two articles in *The New Age* on the introduction of ARV services in prisons.[16] While the coverage acknowledges that many prisoners are living with HIV, it neglects to address HIV risk in prisons that would also necessitate HIV-*prevention* services (in addition to treatment) among incarcerated populations.

Another article in the *Daily Sun* gives a rather graphic account of how a group of high-school boys (for a small fee) will help their schoolmates "jump" male pupils and rape them.[17] The incident has clear MSM connotations and a strong case can be made that the journalist should have addressed the HIV risk inherent in these incidents. Yet these concerns remain unaddressed in the coverage.

Through ongoing advocacy, sexual minorities are being granted increasing recognition in local HIV programmes. Among others, the inclusion of MSM as a "key population" in the new National Strategic Plan goes some way to ensuring these changes are entrenched on a systems level.[18] But although these advances are encouraging, as Van Zyl's journalism suggests, there is still much terrain to be covered. The media will have a prominent part to play in facilitating the acceptance of alternative masculinities and sexualities.

16 Mapumulo, Z. "ARV clinic launched at Leeuwkop Prison", *The New Age* (July 2011); Dube, M. "Taking health care services to prisons", *The New Age* (November 2011).

17 Mokgosi, J. "Boys rape boys for R10", *Daily Sun* (November 2011).

18 SANAC (2011).

References /

Badat, N. (2007) "Out of the closet? But strictly after nine." *IOL news*. Retrieved 2 May 2012, http://www.iol.co.za/news/south-africa/out-of-the-closet-but-strictly-after-nine-1.350606.

Baggaley, RF; White, RG; and Boily, M. (2010) "HIV transmission risk through anal intercourse: Systematic review, meta-analysis and implications for HIV prevention." *International Journal of Epidemiology*, 39, 1048–1063.

Jobson, G. (2010) *HIV prevention for MSM in Cape Town, South Africa: Context, dynamics, recommendations*. Health4Men, Anova Health Institute.

Lane, T; Fisher Raymond, F; Dladla, S; Rosethe, J; Struthers, H; McFarland, W; and McIntyre, J. (2011) "High HIV prevalence among men who have sex with men in Soweto, South Africa: Results from the Soweto Men's Study." *AIDS Behaviour*, 15, 626–634.

Lane, T; Mogale, T; Struthers, H; McIntyre, J; and Kegeles, SM. (2008) "'They see you as a different thing': The experiences of men who have sex with men with healthcare workers in South African township communities." *Sexually Transmitted Infections*, 84, 340–433.

SANAC. (2011) National Strategic Plan on HIV, STIs and TB: 2012–2016.

Sjolund, Y. (2011) "Gay Soweto: New HIV shock." *Health24.com*. Retrieved 2 May 2012, http://www.health24.com/medical/Condition_centres/777-792-814-1768,62076.asp

WHO. (2011) *Guidelines: Prevention and treatment of HIV and other sexually transmitted infections among men who have sex with men and transgender people – recommendations for a public health approach*. World Health Organization, Geneva.

Brokeback marriage

Pieter van Zyl

"Get clean and come back home," was Cecilia's response to her husband Hendrik when he told her he was gay. Like many others, Hendrik's struggle to maintain the façade of family man led him down a path of risky sex and alcohol abuse that left him HIV positive.

Hendrik Viljoen is distracted. It's sticky hot in Durban, unusual for this time of year, yet he hardly notices. For the first time in the six weeks he's spent in rehab, he's being allowed to see his wife.

His hug is restrained, but his 45-year-old wife, Cecilia, doesn't react. He's told her too often in the past decade: she's too fat; he's not attracted to her any more.

This time, he doesn't say it. Instead, he blurts: "All these years, I tried to pin our sexless marriage on you. I have to set the record straight. It's me. I'm gay. That's the only reason we didn't have sex any more – not because I don't love you, not because there is anything wrong with you ..."

Hendrik hears the waves crashing outside. He can smell lunch being prepared. But he knows he won't keep any food down for the rest of the day. Cecilia pulls at a single loose thread on her navy skirt. She cries without making a sound.

She steps toward him. So, he thinks, this is how it will end. He steels himself for a slap. Instead, his wife puts her arms around him.

"I always knew," she says. "But you loved me. You cared for me and the kids. I didn't care. Get clean and come back home."

This is the first time 46-year-old Hendrik has been truly honest with his wife in 25 years.

Cecilia is not unusual in her "Brokeback marriage", the trendy term coined from the Oscar-winning movie of two cowboys who fell in love. A conservative estimate is that 1.7 million to 3.4 million American women are married to men who sleep with other men. In South Africa different groups focusing on the study of sexuality estimate the figure at between 15 and 20 per cent of married men – which works out to about 1.8 million men who have sex with other men.

Like many other young men raised conservatively in small towns, Hendrik married at the age of 21 because "it was the right thing to do". At school he refused to follow the pattern of his openly gay brother, 10 years his senior. "I won't say I was one of the *manne*, but I was definitely not seen as one of the *moffies*. I played rugby, went to parties and had girlfriends at school."

His mom died when he was six and, unable to cope alone with the kids, the boys' father sent them to boarding school in Makhado. "We were four in a room. We played. But there was no mention of being gay! I had three girlfriends at that stage."

Their "playing" bothered Hendrik, though, and he confided in a teacher who told him not to worry. It was completely normal to experiment.

In his matric year, an accident occurred that was to shape his young adult life. Driving with only a learners' licence, he rolled a car and a schoolfriend was killed. Hendrik was in hospital for three months while his leg was reconstructed.

"I still today feel responsible for her death. I was behind the steering wheel. It's me that had to die that day. But I'm alive. I had to start looking for a reason."

After school, he left his small town to work in Pretoria – where he met Cecilia. They clicked. "She made me feel safe. She listened not only to what I said, but what I meant."

Still badly affected by the accident, though, he transferred back to his hometown after only six months. He felt safer living with his sister. By the time he returned to Pretoria, Cecilia was already engaged.

Hendrik was a guest at their wedding. But with an eerie prescience, Cecilia introduced him: "Meet my next husband."

Cecilia's husband died in a car accident two months and 11 days later. She was pregnant. "Our relationship started out as friendship and support in her time of mourning. It, over time, developed into something more romantic."

Hendrik and Cecilia married in 1984 in Pretoria – a month after her son, Carel, was born. Although the spark they shared never flared into passion, he thought their marriage was a good one. In 1987 their daughter, Vanessa, was born.

Hendrik was in Johannesburg for a conference.

"It's me. Do you remember me?" asked a dark man in his early thirties, during morning coffee. He was one of the roommates he'd experimented with in the Makhado hostel.

"Let's get out of here and catch up."

They went for a few drinks and ended up at a Formula 1 Hotel in Midrand. Hendrik had always felt there was something missing from his life, but hadn't been able to put his finger on it. It was there he first experienced a spark of awareness. Both were married, both with two kids. It was the first time either of them had had sex with a man.

Driving home to Ermelo, the doubts churned in Hendrik's head. How could he never have realised what was hidden inside him? He never wanted to see that man again, he decided. And he wouldn't tell his wife, because it would never happen again.

"I was pissed off with myself. We weren't *laaities* any more and should have been able to control our urges. I should have known better. But I thought what my wife and kids didn't know wouldn't hurt them."

Alternative masculinities exist everywhere, though some are more visible than others. For men who have sex with men (MSM) living in townships and informal settlements, being open about their sexuality is often challenging. Widespread stigma and prejudice, and the notion that being homosexual is un-African, often drives them underground and away from safe-sex messages.

But not everyone hides. Lebohang Mashiloane trawled the fringes of male sexuality in South African communities and found a number of remarkable men with the courage to express themselves.

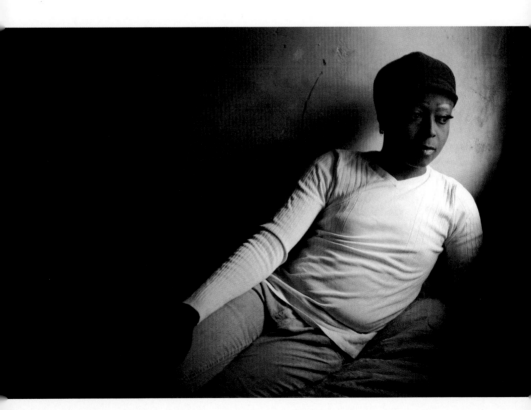

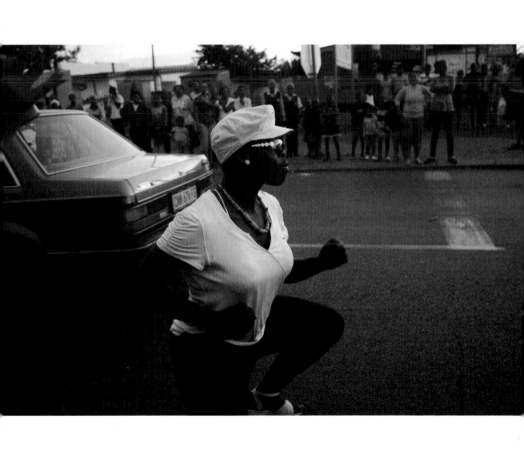

While some men have experienced rejection, others have encoun-
tered less resistance. The introduction of community events such as
Miss Gay Mangaung, in Bochabela township (below), could suggest
a growing tolerance towards alternative expressions of masculinity.

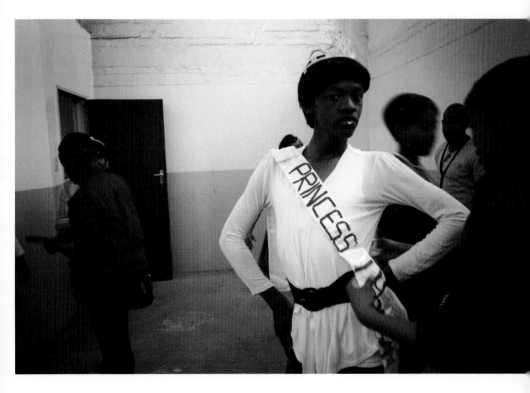

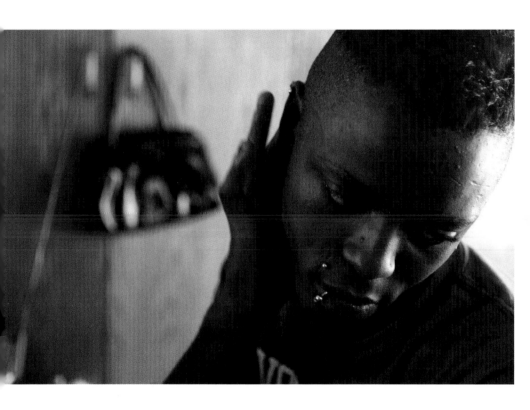

Yet these men continue to exist in a world of uneasy tension between the growing acceptance of alternative masculinities in certain communities and the stigma, discrimination and violence that continue to characterise others.

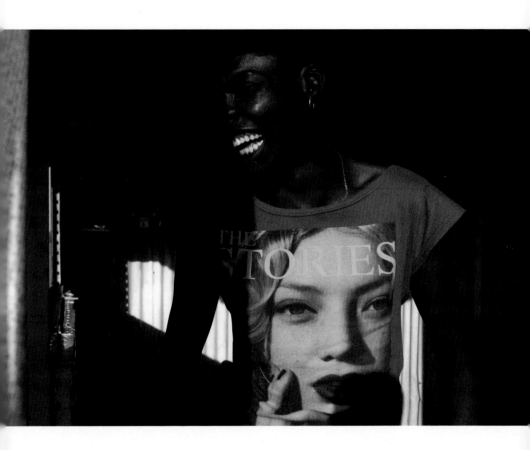

The threat of HIV looms large for MSM, who are biologically already at higher risk of contracting HIV. Added to this is the fact that safe-sex messaging often fails to reach them. Most campaigns addressing men tout heterosexual images and those targeted at openly gay men tend not to speak to all MSM.

Ignorance and stigma in the health sector place the sexual health of these men at even greater risk. While some effort has been made at sensitising healthcare workers and making them more "sex-positive", hostility remains extremely prevalent, putting countless men off seeking critically important sexual health care.

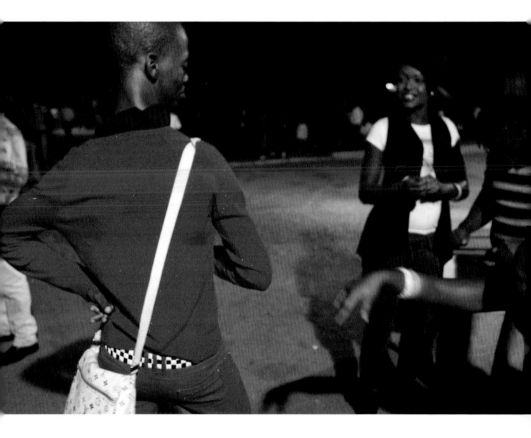

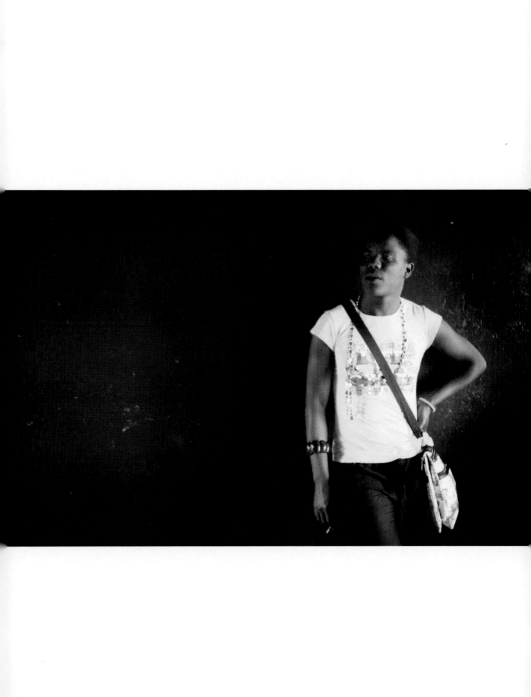

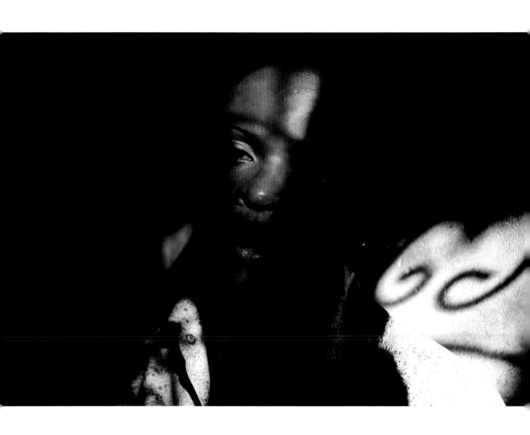

Sexual minorities have received increasing recognition in national planning for HIV treatment and prevention, as exemplified by their inclusion in the latest National Strategic Plan. But much of the change will need to come from within communities and from the healthcare workers themselves, based on a deeper understanding that there is more than one kind of man.

He never saw the other man again. "It was easy for me to make him the scapegoat; that if it wasn't for him, I would never have done this."

Hendrik joined an evangelical congregation in Ermelo. He wanted his demons exorcised. He fought his sexual awakening with every molecule of his being.

"I never spoke to the pastor about it. But every time he called on people who wanted to be prayed for, I went to the front of the church to be saved. God allowed me to stray. He should help me get back to the straight and narrow."

Nonetheless, two months after his first gay experience, it happened again. In Johannesburg on business, he had oral sex in a public toilet. The same feelings of guilt pursued him all the way home.

Hendrik increasingly found excuses to leave Ermelo and hook up with men in the cities. After one particular weekend of gay club-hopping in 1997, Hendrik decided never to have sex with his wife again.

"I felt dirty. I couldn't take what I was doing home. I thought up any reason not to have sex with Cecilia. I told her she was too fat. I told her she wasn't attractive to me any more. I put all the blame on her to hide what I was."

Cecilia was devastated. Oddly, this bothered Hendrik less than telling his family the truth. Only his brother knew. "He was very angry with me. He said I should never have married, because he always knew I was gay. He still blames himself that he did not kick me out the closet earlier."

Thinking he could start afresh, Hendrik moved the family to Durban. "I thought I'd have more time to spend with my family. We would go to the beach and do things together." But after only a few weeks, he realised the city held even more opportunities to live out his fantasies. He visited the steam baths over his lunch hour and on Saturdays – and was pulled deeper and deeper into the gay scene.

"I met other married men visiting these places and slowly but surely did not feel as guilty … I was never too drunk to not know what I was doing. And at that stage, seven years back, I did not care if I was infected with HIV. I felt I deserved AIDS. I already felt infected by being gay. If I died, I might as well die from AIDS. It should be my punishment."

Hendrik began drinking heavily. But after a close call with the police, he was determined never again to drive drunk. He also decided never again to be led into temptation in the arms of another man.

"I knew when I had this drink I wouldn't get into my car and go anywhere. I finished a bottle of whisky a night. It also gave me a reason not to have sex with my wife."

As a brake on his gay activities, it didn't work. He still hooked up with men during the day or after work on Saturdays. The more he cheated on his wife, the less he cared about it.

Eventually though, he was forced to face his alcohol abuse – for the sake of his children. They fled the house when he was drunk and wouldn't bring friends home.

In December 2004 he booked himself into rehab. There he was forced to face his life sober. It was there he had to face the reality: he was gay. It was the first time he had said it out aloud.

And it was there that he tested HIV positive.

His status didn't shock him. "I convinced myself I deserved it. And at that stage I was so focused on becoming alcohol free, I was so tired of the whole process, that my HIV status was shifted back to the back of my mind until I had more energy to deal with it."

Nonetheless he found it too difficult to tell his family he was positive – although he did pluck up the courage to tell his children he was gay. His daughter readily offered her support and affirmed her love. His son accepted the news with more difficulty. "Whatever," he said.

They tried to pick up their lives – to be a family again. But a day after their daughter turned 24, Hendrik told Cecilia he was leaving and wanted a divorce.

Hendrik met Petrus Wessels (49) in cyberspace and they e-mailed for weeks before they met. But the first night they spent together just felt right.

After leaving rehab, he'd taken a second test for insurance purposes. This time Hendrik had tested negative. He had realised his viral load might be too low to be detected, yet he really wanted to believe it. "With my whole heart."

When he fell in love with Petrus, Hendrik tested again. Positive.

His brother was furious. "Maybe you would have been negative if you made peace with who you were earlier," he told Hendrik. But Petrus didn't turn away from him.

Hendrik's two biggest fears are that Cecilia and his children should discover his status, and that he might infect Petrus. "What freaks me out is that he is willing to take chances, but I won't ever play Russian roulette with others' and my own life again. I will be as safe as safe can be ..."

Names have been changed. First published on health24.com *on 23 August 2010.*

After nine at Bra Mo's

Pieter van Zyl

In the safety of a small dwelling, in an informal settlement on the outskirts of Cape Town, men gather to be themselves and to love who they please – each other.

The Cape Flats are cold and wet, but it's warm and welcoming in Bra Mo's place in Crossroads. From outside a faint glow is visible through a slit in the curtains. A stack of empty bottles lies near the front door.

But as the door opens, laughter and shrieks of excitement spill the life that is inside out over the pavement.

"Hola! I'm just fetching more chairs from next door," 52-year-old Mo explains while rushing past into the rain. When he returns, another five men have arrived. Mo runs out again.

For the rest of the evening, men come and go, sometimes disappearing two at a time into one of the two small bedrooms in the back.

It's not easy being gay in the township. Mo is seen as the big daddy, the "queer mother" of Crossroads. He provides a space for them to be themselves.

"To us – we who have to look out for each other's well-being," Mo says, lifting his glass. "May no one here ever get sick or die alone ..."

Bra Mo's home in Crossroads is a few blocks from the clinic where an HIV vaccine is being tested. He works as an administrator at a clinic in the area and dishes out advice to his guests, along with food and drink.

Mo's house rules are very clear. A framed, handwritten wooden sign a few inches above the TV reads: "*Ndincede mutakwethu yenza ozokuyenza apha kuba enyenenye. Ayifuni wena itsho into khululeka.*" Loosely translated it means: "This is my house, don't judge what I'm doing." Another sign tells guests that the owner of this place has aims and objectives. And that higher powers are always visiting – God the Father and the ancestors: "*Imizamo yam yophela ndakuti ka kuwe.*"

Bra Mo's door is always open.

It's 10 am when Mo opens the door, Black Label quart in hand.

"Come in. They don't allow me to sleep. I'm so tired. But I can't miss out on anything."

Bra Mo says he has known he was gay "since that photograph was taken". He gestures at a framed, black-and-white photograph of himself at 16. "But at that time I couldn't say anything. Men don't do these things. But as young boys we sometimes had to sleep very close together at our homes in Cathcart. And then we did do something."

He worked as a policeman in Tilden for eight years. In that time he got married to a police clerk. "She was 16 when I met her." They were married for 12 years and had two sons before he fell in love with a nurse and followed her to Cape Town. But she left him when she caught him in bed with a young man.

"She was broken. I won't ever forget her face there in the door-way. I don't want to forget that face. No other woman I care for should ever look like that again."

Over lunch, Mabhuti Mkangeli (36) arrives. He is a respected, soft-spoken gay activist from Lower Crossroads who works at the Triangle Project. He is just explaining the concept of MSM (men having sex with men), when two young men arrive in a blue Mazda.

"They love having sex with gays," someone announces, gesturing at the newcomers just before they walk in.

Fani (30) kisses Mabuthi on the lips as he enters and sits down across from him. His friend Tsepo (24) sits on the floor in front of the TV watching Leon Shuster's *You Must Be Joking*.

"We know you are *moffies*, but we feel comfortable here. You are good to us," says Fani to the men at Mo's.

"And if I like to be on my own, I sit and watch TV," Tsepo adds. "No one bugs me, no one pushes me to do something I don't want to."

Mo, who slipped out earlier, now arrives back with another bootload of beers. "See how nice it is here?" Tsepo exclaims.

When pressured to explain what they get from sex with men, or if they are in fact "straight", the two men clam up. "That's something private!"

"It's a problem," Ronnie Ngalo (44), a respected community leader, explains. "Men having sex with men do not like to use condoms. It makes the experience less pleasant, they say. And then they go back to their wife or girlfriend who asks: 'Why do you want to wear a condom if you only have sex with me?' This is why these men also don't use condoms – to not make their wives suspicious."

Mabhuti steers clear of men with wives and girlfriends. "As a gay activist, I don't want to be part of that stigma that gay men want to turn all straight men gay. I keep to openly gay lovers."

Thursday is big party night in the townships.

"We call it *Hlamba izipaji*. Washing of wallets. People are drinking to prepare for the party of the weekend," Sammi (29), one of Mo's neighbours, explains.

Again, there are no women in sight.

"Sho, sho, sho! It will lead to catfights," Ronnie chimes in.

"We have sex with men [but] we say it's our friends," Sammi adds.

"Some of their wives know, others don't know, some will fight back ... I'm from Gugulethu. My sister is a nurse and accepts me as a gay man, but the rest of the family don't know. My lover stays with his parents in a *hokkie* in the backyard. There we can meet alone."

Sammi walks over to a man hidden in the corner and hugs him. "This is my lover. He is a teacher at a school here nearby."

Buthi (37) is the big, silent type. He wears a long, black, leather trench coat and sits in the corner dragging on a long beaded pipe, usually reserved for the elders in Xhosa villages.

In the late afternoon Themba (37) makes an entrance no one can ignore.

"On Saturdays I'm gay and do boys. On Sundays I'm playing straight and go for girls," he sings with a Savanna in one hand.

He's a lecturer at a Cape Town university and has a 15-year-old son. "He looks like me. But my son is stubborn. And he has a big problem with my lifestyle. He will tell me: 'Please don't talk like that, don't do that. I'm fed up with your gayness.'"

Themba's partner is Victor (23), a young Usher-lookalike behind trendy sunglasses. They met four months ago at Rosie's in De Water-kant.

"I like him because he's so self-assured. When he asked me to get married, it felt like a good idea at the time."

The two are engaged, although men hover constantly around Victor, forcing Themba to intervene frequently. Victor stays in Philippi with his aunt and works as waiter in Cape Town.

"To move in with Themba in Wynberg? Not yet. We have to be very sure before I do that. But it's difficult to be myself staying with the family."

At this point, Themba announces: "The Constitution protects my rights. I have the right to drink this. I have the right to love this man ... We grew up in such a restricted society. When we come out the closet, we fall out. You will know I'm gay. I'll make sure of that."

At Phuga's restaurant and pub in Gugulethu, Bra Mo and friends have just finished an afternoon of drinking. They had a braai at the world-renowned Mzoli's next door and are walking back to his place.

It's Saturday afternoon and, in at least three houses within a block, people have gathered under tents for funeral services.

"We lost five friends to AIDS, but we only found that out after they were buried. They had to die alone," Mo laments. "You never really know how many of your friends are busy dying of this sickness. There is still a huge stigma here in the township."

In the front yard of one of the new houses in White City, Nyanga, a family is slaughtering chickens – five feathered corpses already lie to one side waiting to be boiled in a pot. In the graveyard nearby, kids are playing cricket among the tombstones. Life and death live side by side here.

A car drives by: "*Molweni moffies*," the drunk youngsters shout.

"Ag, we know," Mo shouts back. "Tonight. After nine we'll see you. You will come knocking on my door!"

Some names have been changed. Originally published on health24.com *on 23 August 2010.*

Loxion–Boy pride

Pieter van Zyl

*He's chosen life in the colourful townships and expresses his alter-
native sexuality with confidence and flair. White and Afrikaans-
speaking, Frik blurs the lines that are sometimes harshly drawn in
South African society.*

The huge machine comes into action, steely tentacles printing
T-shirts with iconic township images – young men swanking in
fancy clothes, R5-a-trip Toyota *amaphelas* (taxis), a Black Label beer
bottle, a train steaming into Heideveld station, a two-plate stove …

The 45-year-old artist may not have been born to these images,
but he has grown to embrace them. George Frederick Myburgh is
known to his friends in the suburbs as Frik. In the township, he is
called Mister Fred or Mister George by his neighbours.

In a still-divided country, in which white and black live largely
apart, Frik decided to keep his life as simple as his designs – and to
spend it in the townships. In Gugulethu, where he works at the Cape
Town College's Gugulethu campus, Frik is just another of the few
hundred thousand people who live and work in the township. An
Afrikaner *boerseun* with a native heart. He pays R200 a month rent
and grows his own vegetables and herbs as he had done with his dad
on their Northern Cape farm.

He pulls at the woollen cap covering his close-shaven head. A
thick, black jacket warms this aesthete's body. "I've been living on
and off in townships for almost two decades. I see myself as a Loxion
Boy, as someone living by the philosophy of the location – keeping
life simple; being happy with what you've got."

"Even those Loxion Boys driving flashy cars, still stop to eat an *igwinya* and go to shebeens."[19]

For lunch Frik eats a R1 *igwinya* with *slap tjips* (fries) he orders from the campus takeaway, run by his landlady. He has been staying in her house in Gugs for the last six months. In NY6. The NY denotes Native Yard – a reminder of apartheid, which stands in stark contrast to the meaning of Gugulethu: Xhosa for "Our Pride".

At Frik's home, late afternoon, there is a buzz of visitors and house music. He is busy in his tin shack studio in the back, creating bold crayon drawings and paintings of township life, using paper potato bags as canvases.

His backyard is divided into a quilt of small herb patches and flower beds fenced off by empty glass bottles buried top down in the ground.

"This one I christened *Kleinplasie*. That one is *Dawidspan*." Frikkie points towards each painting and calls out its name: "*Duurwater*. It was my grandfather's farm between Douglas and Griekwastad, where he had to struggle pumping the water from the dam on top of the Ghaapse mountains. And that one is *Perdekloof* ... These are all the farms of people I knew."

Frik loves to sit in his kraal and smoke with his beer a hand's-width away. Here you can drink, chat, make music to your heart's

---

19   An *igwinya* is a type of doughnut, also known as a *vetkoek* in Afrikaans and a shebeen is a township pub.

content. "My friends and I, we're too noisy for the suburbs."

His kitchen exudes a rural charm. Here he prepares real traditional Afrikaner fare, known as *boerekos*: thick meat soup, roasted vegetables, rice and a rustic chicken pie with the meat still on the bone bubbling under the homemade crust. His speciality is malva pudding, mom's recipe.

He dishes up on antique crockery, heirlooms from his parent's farm, Modderrivier. Tonight his guests will feast on dishes that are virtually the same as those served at his parents' house the night he came out.

Frik was born in 1963 to an average Afrikaner family, but one that allowed him to choose his friends and mix with whom he liked. He was brought up in Douglas, a small Northern Cape town nestled in between the great Orange and Vaal rivers. He went to school in Warrenton.

"I have hands like my mom's," Frik remarks. "We have the same long fingers."

His dad was mayor of Douglas for years, a businessman with a butchery. But in the early 1970s he went bankrupt and had to start selling off some of his property. Thankfully, his dad knew how to spot opportunities. He heard about an auction of 60 pigs no one wanted and he picked up the animals for a song.

With all the pigs, the soil on the farm was enriched. They started selling super-sized vegetables to people in the township outside Warrenton. They did so well, his dad bought more land and started a fresh-produce market.

Frik inherited his dad's creativity and decided to complete a national diploma in textile design at the Pretoria Technikon. After that, he took charge of a tapestry and weaving centre in Bushbuck-ridge, in the old homeland of Lebowa, on the north-eastern boundary of South Africa.

"There I got my first taste of township life."

In 1989 he moved back to the farm outside Kimberley. He found work as a production manager of a big clothing factory in town.

It was in the middle of the winter of 1990 that his parents invited Frik to come over for dinner. His mom seldom uses his nickname, but when she does, he knows she's up to something. "Kadool, please come home to Modderrivier, we want to speak to you."

It was a Wednesday night and bitterly cold. But his parents greeted him with the same warmth and love he was used to. The three of them held hands to say grace, as always, before they ate in silence.

After malva pudding, when the plates were cleared away, Frik's dad jumped right in: "Your brother said you are now 'that way'. What do you want us to do? Should we send you to a psychologist or get the *dominee* to talk to you? Should we do something to help?"

"No, please. This is my life. I don't want to go and see anyone. I don't want to change," was his reply.

And that was that. The subject was laid to rest. No one mentioned it again until years later, after his dad had died of Alzheimer's. Frik and his mom would sometimes chat about his sexuality. But she was never nosy – even when he had a black lover.

He met Thulani, or Mr T, on a Friday afternoon in Queen's

Park, Kimberley's favourite cruising spot for gay men. Frik had just returned from two years working in a restaurant on the Isle of Man. It was the turn of the new century.

Frik immediately spotted the tall, strongly built man sitting on one of the park benches. When he returned from the UK, he idly wondered what it would be like to have a long-term black boyfriend. So, hell, why not?

When their eyes met, the man waved him over. It was broad daylight and a public place, but he had long ago stopped worrying what people thought of him.

Thulani was Zimbabwean. He had just turned 26 and was struggling to find work. Frik suggested they start up a business together until something better came along. They were together for 10 years.

From the day they met, Thulani drove Frik everywhere in Frik's dad's bakkie. Thulani gave Frik a passion for township life. They went to shebeens together and met an array of colourful characters. Together they opened a shop in Galeshewe, outside Kimberley. The shop sold vegetables and Frik's art.

When Frik decided to try out the Western Cape, Thulani followed. They rented a garage next to a house in Langa for "next to nothing". Frik converted it into a home. His favourite place became the roof, where he sat looking out over the township and drawing what he saw.

There they started a spaza shop, selling little bags of sweets and loose cigarettes, packets of flour and so on. Thulani got work on building sites.

But things eventually turned sour. Thulani met a girlfriend and Frik was worried that he was sleeping around without protection. It was time to end the relationship.

Thulani was reluctant to go. It was only when Frik handed Mr T the keys for his father's bakkie that he disappeared forever from his life.

Nearly two years later, when Frik was in his early thirties, James walked into his life. Frik had just returned from another trip to England and went for a stroll on the Sea Point promenade. He felt liberated, and wasn't keen to start a new relationship. James was working the promenade as a "rent piece", a sex worker.

Frik sat down on a bench beside him, looking out over the waves. They started chatting and connected. When he discovered what James did for a living, Frik helped him get off the streets by organising him a job as a restaurant gardener.

On 1 February 2002 James was thrown from a train after being robbed of his cellphone. He broke his neck and back. During the last few weeks of his life, Frik visited James in hospital every day, rubbing Vaseline into his feet, telling him to keep on fighting.

But he died exactly two months after the accident. Frik was on his own again.

Here in Gugulethu Frik has found his soul. He is optimistic that he might someday find love again.

Yesterday he planted some rose-scented geraniums in his *imtlanti* (kraal) in the back. It's a reminder to himself of a time when his grief and solitude nearly drove him to take his own life in the Swartberg Pass near Prince Albert.

"The scent now reminds me to live."

He will never move back to the suburbs, though. "When I retire, I'll buy a house in Khayelitsha and move there."

Don't let me be misunderstood

Pieter van Zyl

"And now that you're sure you are gay, I have to inform you that I'm carrying your child." Since he heard those words from his girlfriend, Ronnie has come a long way, to gay activist, exemplary community member and HIV-positive role model.

In a cul-de-sac in the heart of Elsiesrivier, people are pouring into the street. The mood is festive. It's a memorial service for Ronnie Ngalo's uncle, who died in an accident six years ago.

"We are saying our farewell to my Uncle Lukas," Ronnie explains. "After today his wife and family do not have to mourn any more."

Today, 44-year-old Ronnie is not the activist for children's rights, the outspoken gay man from Nyanga. Today he is an important link in the Ngalo family's ritual to appease the ancestors. Later, however, when the other men are in the front yard eating, drinking and chatting, Ronnie feels more comfortable in the lounge.

"As the gay man in the family, this is how I often feel. Neither here nor there."

On the way to Ronnie's place in White City, Nyanga, the *phela* (township taxi) pumps and grinds to the beat of the hip hop hit by Lil Wayne: "Oh Lord, please don't let me be misunderstood ..."

Everyone knows his home as a safe house, a place for the queer at heart to come and relax. Here Ronnie provides shelter for the lonely, for gay lovers who can't be intimate in their overcrowded family homes, for the old and the scared. Ronnie sits with friends outside the "wendy house", as Ronnie prefers to call his prefabricated home.

"Thank God it's not raining!"

When more guests arrive, Ronnie disappears inside and returns with a plate of muffins. "I baked these myself. It's my mom's recipe." He loves feeding people. Almost every afternoon, you'll find him on the pavement in front of his house, braaiing and selling meat to passers-by.

Even with tongs in hand, sweating over the flames, Ronnie is stylishly dressed: pin-striped pants, crisp white shirt, waistcoat, a colourful scarf and his trademark woollen peaked cap.

A woman walks over and it transpires Ronnie was a mentor for her troubled son. "If it wasn't for you he would have been in Pollsmoor [prison]. Thank you!"

A few hours later two women with babies on their backs arrive to pay back loans. "When we struggle with money, we can always come here," one explains. "The day my boyfriend gets paid I bring the money back."

Ronnie shrugs: "They have babies. They have to eat. I don't always get it back. But it's fine. I'm never hungry or lonely."

As airplanes crisscross overhead on their way to and from Cape Town International, people come and go. Every half-hour, there's a new face joining the "gay bash".

"I also call it BOBs: Bring your Own Bottle," says Ronnie. His dream is to open a gay shebeen in the township. "A place where everyone will feel at home: gay and straight."

When and if he finally gets his RDP house, he will keep the "wendy house" and run it as a shebeen, a shelter or a soup kitchen. Inside, he has made his house a home. One wall is covered in African trinkets and, on another, photographs of Ronnie with different hair-styles: dreadlocks, cropped, *bleskop* (bald). The TV blares soapies.

Next to his bed a row of "luxury skin products" from an overseas hotel stand ready to be used. Condoms and lube lie in wait next to Fred Khumalo's *Bitches' Brew*.

Two elderly ladies arrive and Ronnie fetches beers from the fridge. "I'm part of their *stokvel*," says Ronnie. "I pay between R200 and R500 each month. And by the end of the year we each get our share."

Until recently Ronnie worked for the Molo Songololo Child & Human Rights organisation as Youth Programmes coordinator. He has just started as coordinator for an AIDS management programme in Claremont. He is a board member of Triangle Project and a trustee of the Pride Shelter Trust. He belongs to his area's community policing forum and is part of the street committee.

Ronny Ngalo is a community leader.

His most vivid teen memory is when he had his first alcoholic drink. A tot of Clubman Mint Punch. Ronnie was 19 and walking with his uncle for two hours from the Zwelethemba township to the place in the "bush" at Aan de Doorns. Ronnie's cousin was being initiated in the Xhosa tradition. The effect of the alcohol almost allowed him to come out to Uncle Wilson, with whom he had a better relationship than his dad. But he was not ready yet.

Ronnie's initiation and traditional circumcision were in 1986 – also at Aan de Doorns. This time all his uncles were there to make sure he was okay.

"Everyone was concerned about me like a delicate egg."

Ronnie was chosen as part of the first group of five boys to get the knife. The elders thought he was ready.

"It was a big achievement to finish before your time. Everyone was proud of me."

"When there is any sign that a Xhosa boy might be gay, he is sent to the bush to be circumcised and initiated into manhood as soon as possible. When this boy comes back and is still gay, he moves to the city to be able to live his life."

Ronnie was born on 14 June 1964 in Worcester and grew up in a coloured community. "I think it is much less judgmental than the Transkei where my dad, William, is from." But he does remember, when he was 15, a man told his parents: "He's a funny boy. He's too much like a woman."

"During break, boys would chase me around and try to bully me and steal my lunch. By the age of 13 I was already a panic-button person like I'm now. If there is injustice, I report it. I always reported these bullies to the teachers."

In his twenties, all but one of his siblings knew he was gay and accepted it.

But his eldest brother did not even want to speak to him.

"It's not part of the Xhosa tradition to be gay. You're not a woman, you are a man!"

They did not speak for years. Eventually though, they sat down together and Ronnie explained that he was not hurting himself, or anyone around him. His brother calmed down then, but still took a while to truly accept him. Four months after their reconciliation, his brother phoned to invite Ronnie to a cleansing ceremony at his new house in Delft.

"I had to perform the duties of the man of the house. I had to speak to the elders. I had to help slaughter the sheep. My brother made me a very important part of his life."

It was when he was studying to be a teacher in Worcester that Ronnie met the mother of his son.

"I didn't like the idea of sleeping with a woman, but through peer pressure I started to go out with her. In those days homosexual teachers were frowned upon."

She regularly accompanied him to school functions. "I just had to play that role of being straight."

Then a friend of hers spotted Ronnie at a gay party in Khayelitsha and she confronted him about it.

"What you hear is true," Ronnie said. "I was wrong not to tell you."

"And now that you're sure you are gay," she replied, "I have to inform you that I'm carrying your child."

Ronnie was torn between shock and excitement. Until that moment he had never thought of being a father.

"Please, please don't shut me out of this child's life," Ronnie begged. "I will provide for him. I will make sure he has money for education."

Ronnie is grateful she realised the child would want a father in his life, even if he is gay.

"My son has just turned 15 and often comes to visit. He is very straight. That's why he doesn't feel threatened by all the gay men here at my house. But we never discuss my sexuality. He's at a very difficult age at the moment and I try to protect him from my issues."

His son is a good sportsman. "I'm so proud. He did not get that from his dad."

In 1984 Ronnie moved from Wellington to Cape Town "for greener pastures".

"In those years we were so scared of being discovered in the townships."

Ronnie and his friends frequented a gay-friendly and "black-friendly" nightclub called Tots in Long Street. There they met a well-to-do tea farmer from the old Transkei. When it got too late to go home to the township, they stayed with him in Green Point.

"I still remember that white woman, one of his neighbours in the block of flats, screaming: 'Here comes a flock of black *moffies*'. She phoned the police and our friend had to bribe the police not to arrest us."

He met his first long-term lover in 1987. Ronnie stayed with Marco for 10 years, moving with him to Port Elizabeth. They had a house in Lorraine and tried not to make it too obvious that a mixed-race, gay couple was building a life together just next door.

But in 2001 Marco suddenly died of a heart attack.

"The bottom of my world fell out," Ronnie remembers. He was left with a Ford Cortina that Marco bought for him in Mossel Bay in the 1980s. He sold the car and used the money to buy the "wendy house", where he still stays.

Ronnie has now been living with HIV for almost five years. His most recent CD4 count was 225. A healthy person's is between 800 and a thousand. His viral load is undetectable.

"I feel great! I take my medication every day."

He tested at the Christiaan Barnard Memorial Hospital in Cape Town in March 2005 during Gay Pride. He'd been losing a lot of weight and had constant stomach cramps. "I was at a Pride function in Sea Point and the pain got so bad I could not even stand up straight."

He ended up in hospital. During those three days a nurse suggested they do a series of tests, including a screening for HIV.

Three weeks after he was discharged, he went back for his results. "When I heard the word 'positive' I felt so weak. When I arrived home, I got into bed and slept the rest of the day. For three days I did not want to go anywhere."

But his friends refused to allow him to slip deeper into depression. He was invited to a house party in Crossroads and was pulled – kicking and screaming – back into life again.

He was put on ARVs and here he is, still going strong.

"I love life," he says simply.

Some names have been changed.

My crusade against HIV

Pieter van Zyl

It started with a skin rash that looked like eczema. His heels cracked and started bleeding ... In 2009 local soapie star Renaldo Adams learned that he was HIV positive. Now he is helping others come to terms with their status and live healthily with HIV.

A man dashes up the stairs into the offices of Health4Men, a men's health and treatment organisation in De Waterkant, Cape Town.

"I need to get tested. Please!" He seems desperate.

Renaldo Adams (38), a field worker for Health4Men, explains very calmly: "I'm able to assist you."

Renaldo hates being panic-stricken himself. That's why one of his missions is to restore calm around him as soon as possible. He knows what this man is going through. An HIV test a few months ago also changed his life.

His work at Health4Men was his saving grace. Through the darkest place in his life, he started working with others.

"It gives me a sense of redemption, of satisfaction."

Renaldo is part of a team doing research in the townships on how to spread the safe-sex message in the gay community there.

Until recently Renaldo was better known as a *skollie* in *Egoli*, the popular CIA agent known as "The Shadow" in *Interrogation Room* and a Xhosa-speaking doctor in SABC2's soapie *Montana*. But now Renaldo has become a poster boy for living positively with HIV.

The phones in the Health4Men office ring off the hook.

Research has shown that gay men are reluctant to get tested. "If I don't test positive I'm negative," it's believed. It's this head-in-the-sand mentality that needs to be challenged. Renaldo has been part of this change. Every time a man, like the rain-soaked Johannesburg truck driver who just came in, walks in to get tested, he considers it a small victory.

In the not-too-distant past he was obsessed with flashy cars, label clothes and designer furniture. He drove a BMW 320 and an Audi A4. When he bought presents, he made sure the recipient knew it was from a boutique.

These days he is quite happy with his blue Chicco Golf and the dogs in the back. When he brings gifts, it's likely to be a pot of his speciality curry or a bunch of flowers. He has come a long way.

Renaldo was born and grew up in the small town of Butterworth in the former Transkei. He and his family stayed in the so-called coloured township: two rows of houses where almost everyone was related.

He was a small and sensitive boy, teased by his big brothers for being a *moffie*. Growing up with five brothers made him strong, though, and prepared him to deal with bullies at school.

"There was no malice when his brothers teased him," remembers Shirley Adams, Renaldo's sister-in-law and confidante. "He was a difficult boy to understand. He had his way of thinking and doing things. He was the youngest in the home. To tease is what older brothers do."

He and his mom, Frances Adams, were very close. Renaldo was the *laatlammetjie*, born much later than his other siblings. He had a different father from his 10 brothers and sisters. But they never referred to him as their half-brother.

"I never felt like an outsider at home. Even though my birth was the result of a hit-and-run encounter between my mom and dad."

Everyone fussed over Renaldo. "He was terribly spoilt," remembers Shirley. "The whole family liked to dress up nicely. His mom always dressed like a lady with pencil heels on. I remember the first time I met Renaldo at the age of 10, he was wearing a black velvet suit. He wore it to all the important occasions."

For as long as Renaldo could remember, Frances had to look after five daughters and six sons by herself. With only Grade 8, she first worked as a cleaner at a hotel. But was determined to up-skill herself as a homeopath.

"She was such a free spirit. She had no husband and didn't have to answer to anyone," Renaldo remembers. "With a role model like that, I really don't know why I've been so self-obsessed for a big part of my life."

His mother died in 1983 from complications after a gallstone operation. Renaldo was 13 and inconsolable.

Renaldo realised he was gay during puberty. He went to high school in East London and stayed with a very strict uncle. His sexuality was never discussed, but Shirley had a hunch. He was different from other boys and that endeared him to her.

"Renaldo loved those wide Punjabi yoga pants. He sewed himself a pair. But he also wanted a pair of pink pants."

In Grade 9 she bought him a pair, as well as a cropped red top for Christmas. "He loved it. I allowed him to be who he wanted to be."

Shirley was the first person he came out to. It was during the study break before his final matric exams.

"Shirley, I'm gay. I'm certain about it."

He asked her to call his brother Peter into the room – before he lost his nerve. But as Peter walked in, Renaldo broke down and sobbed. The fear of being rejected by his big bother was too much.

Renaldo ran from the house and only returned after dark.

"We love you, we will be here to support you," Shirley promised when he returned. Peter was a man of few words, but it was he who got books from the library about being gay for Renaldo to read. He brought the priest to chat to Renaldo about his sexuality and about how important it was to love himself as he was.

In time the rest of the family also chose the route of acceptance.

After seven years' working as a flight attendant, Renaldo came to earth in Cape Town where he met his first boyfriend and found work as an actor. He was always aware of the dangers of HIV. That was why he preferred long-term relationships.

Just a year ago Renaldo did not know anyone who was openly HIV positive. He thought it better not to know. But in the back of his mind he knew there were those few, rare casual sexual encounters.

It started with skin rash that looked like eczema. His heels cracked and started bleeding. His lungs felt as heavy as lead. He was constantly short of breath.

But then, it could just be TB, couldn't it? And that was curable.

"I became very absent-minded. It felt as though I was losing my mind. I started to forget where I put things and where I should meet people and what time we agreed on. I was constantly tired and just wanted to sleep. There had to be some reason for this."

The answer was at the end of the needle. In December 2009 he went to a clinic in Parklands. His previous test had been five years back. At the clinic his finger was pricked and within 15 minutes he knew his status ...

It was a Friday evening when Shirley got the call.

"I got tested," Renaldo told her. Before he said anything else she knew he had tested HIV positive. She had been worried about his weight loss.

She wept. The first thing that came to mind was that this was a death sentence to this man she loved so much. But she had been trained as an AIDS counsellor by the bank where she was manager. That helped her put the news into perspective.

"I knew I had to be strong and pull myself together."

Shortly after his screening, Renaldo felt like he was contaminated and dying. His CD4 count was 61. A healthy person's count is anything from 800 to a thousand.

"I felt like giving up and fading away."

But when Shirley arrived from Somerset West, she came prepared. The only way for Renaldo to recover was to put on weight.

"Give him a Power Sandwich and Egg Flip shakes," she was instructed by her in-laws from the Eastern Cape. She arrived with powdered milk, baby porridge, eggs, vanilla essence and peanut butter. By the time the rest of the family heard of his status and came over, they thought Shirley had exaggerated. By then he was on ARVs and looked well again.

"You have to spread this message of hope," Shirley told him.

Originally published in Drum *magazine on 7 January 2010.*

Loving a man with HIV

Pieter van Zyl

The lives of a gay couple are forever changed after a night in a holding cell leaves one of them HIV positive.

On his thirty-fifth birthday Wynand Griesel, inebriated from one too many celebratory drinks, got behind the wheel. He ended up behind bars in Sea Point police station for the first few hours of what should have been a happy birthday. Standing in his cell, the only thing he could think about was how he could get off the hook.

Outside dawn was breaking. On the cell wall, he could just barely decipher "Nice to kill", scratched into the powder-blue paint with a fingernail. "Next time, think," someone had written centimetres away, while a faint message on the opposite wall read: "My wish was to be happy and try to start over."

While Wynand tried to keep his mind occupied, his partner Neil Strydom (42), was locked in another holding cell, desperately trying not to lose his mind and to live through the pain.

"Time heals," was just visible to Neil, scratched into the wall in front of him. But he kept repeating it while seven co-detainees took turns raping him.

The situation in the country's prisons and holding cells are a direct public health issue, experts have warned. In its latest report, the organisation Just Detention International paints a gloomy picture, saying the way people are detained has a direct link to the country's HIV epidemic.

The prevalence in South African jails and holding cells is twice that of the infection in the general public. By not preventing sexual violence amongst detainees, the government is in effect sentencing people to death before they have even been found guilty of anything.

Neil was locked up an hour after Wynand – for interfering with a police officer. They wanted to "calm him down" after Wynand's arrest, shut him up.

"*Jou mond is mos lekker los* [You've got a big mouth]. Let's see what happens to someone like you. We'll speak tomorrow," the policeman had told him.

As soon as he entered the cell, he knew he was in trouble. He could smell it in the damp and in the detainees' sweat. The police removed his belt and rings, but he still had a silver bracelet. The officer hadn't spotted it, but one of the men in the cell had.

"If you give it to me, I'll protect you," the faceless voice whispered, when the door had clanged and the cell was submerged in darkness. Neil handed it over.

"We are going to fuck you 'til you bleed," one of the other detainees growled. Someone grabbed his arms and ripped at his clothes.

"Don't fight." There was no chance of that. Neil's 42-year-old, 60-kilogram body was no match for the men. They took turns tearing him open. He stopped counting after the seventh man took over. He tried to focus on something else, but he felt the blood trickling down the inside of his leg.

He screamed, but no one came. A policeman later joked that if they had to open a cell every time someone screamed, they wouldn't get any sleep.

Raindrops trickled down the pub's window. More than three months had passed. Wynand was waiting patiently for almost an hour for Neil to open up and tell him the result of the test. He had gone to the doctor on his own, without letting Wynand know.

Neil drained his third Castle draft and stretched his hand across the bar to touch Wynand's. The waves crashed onto the Bantry Bay rocks, throwing up wisps of foam. The sky was a steely grey.

"I'm sorry, so sorry. Forgive me," Neil broke the silence at last. "Please don't leave me. I've tested positive."

After a couple of drinks they walked home, Wynand's arm hooked through Neil's. It smelt clean, with the rain pouring down. Every time Wynand tried to speak, Neil's face became a mask of agony. Wynand was crying, but no one would notice – his face awash with early spring rain. At their flat in Victoria Road he had to carry Neil up the stairs.

"Will you ever touch me again?" Neil asked. "I don't want to infect you."

"I won't leave you. Just give me a chance."

Pulling Neil towards him, trying to envelope him, Wynand added: "I wish I could have protected you. I wish I was there."

They met at a crossroads in both their lives. Neil was still coming to terms with his dad's death from a heart attack. And he had just lost his job, after the owner of his interior design company died of cancer. He was a white, middle-aged man without a job in South Africa.

Wynand was coming to terms with his sexuality. They met at Café Manhattan, a gay-friendly bar and restaurant in De Waterkant, the "pink village".

Wynand did everything possible to resist being drawn deeper into a serious relationship with Neil. But Neil made him feel that he'd been missing out on something. He'd been missing out on his second half.

After the test, Wynand watched for signs of the virus breaking down his lover's body. But all he wanted to see was the smile, and that returned a little more slowly.

Neil noticed that he looked "hollowed out". His body reminded him of death, he said. But it made it easier to know that Wynand loved him.

His feet hurt. They couldn't go on hiking trips, as they'd done before. It was too painful. Peripheral neuropathy made his feet, hands and back to go into spasms. The human immunodeficiency virus (HIV), which causes AIDS, causes extensive damage to the central and peripheral nervous systems. A rapidly progressive, painful polyneuropathy affecting the feet and hands is often the first clinically apparent sign of HIV infection. The pain never goes away.

After work, it became a ritual. Neil would take his socks off and Wynand would massage each toe, the bridge of each foot, each heel.

Eating was laborious for Neil. Once he started ARVs, his appetite became almost non-existent. Wynand kept his bedside table stocked with tempting snacks: nuts, biltong and his favourite soul food, Chipniks.

Safe sex was always an obsession for Wynand. Twice a year he went for an HIV test.

One of the first things Neil noticed about Wynand was the free clinic visitor's card in Wynand's wallet when he paid for a meal.

Until Neil's test result, Wynand had never been close to anyone with the virus. Now he was sleeping with the enemy – and he'd never been happier. The love was more than the fear. But he still got tested every six months – just to make 100 per cent sure.

Every night before getting into bed, Neil sorts four types of medicine into two small heaps of pills – one for that night and one for the morning. One Combivir® tablet in each pile. One Virimune® in each. That takes care of the virus.

Half an Epilim 500® – an anti-psychotic – tonight. The other half tomorrow. And a yellow-and-white Venlor XR 150mg in the morning. An anti-depressant. There are side effects: he lost his appetite, lost 10 kilograms in two years, has constant headaches and feels drained and tired.

Sometimes Neil wonders why he keeps on taking the medicine. Then he repeats his mantra to himself: "You don't want to die. You don't want to die."

Names have been changed.

Separating the boys from the men

The main reason for having sex immediately after initiation is to test if the new "Mercedes Benz" worked effectively. It is also through sex that they rid themselves of extreme bad luck. They believe they should sula, *or wipe it off, by sleeping with someone of "lesser value" than a loved one.*

"We do get a lot of criticism from people saying it is mutilation or that we are like a factory – you can say that if you're living in a country where HIV prevalence is 2 per cent. But if you live in Africa where HIV prevalence is 24 per cent, you cannot brush it off like that."

Separating the boys from
the men / Introduction

Between 2009 and 2010 journalism fellows Mthetho Tshemese and Wilson Johwa, of the HIV & AIDS Media Project, made male circumcision the focus of their research. Tshemese set out to investigate the controversial practice of traditional male circumcision (TMC), while Johwa subsequently came to grips with government's endorsement of medical male circumcision (MMC) as a means to reducing HIV risk. Both produced accounts that make for valuable glimpses into how men regard their masculinity and how this relates to the South African HIV epidemic.

Circumcision literally cuts to the core of masculinity. In the strictly physical and most obvious sense, it is a direct engagement with the key biological marker of manhood – the penis. But there are many, far more nuanced ties between the removal of the foreskin and masculinity. For many cultures it is the watershed between boyhood and being a man. The procedure is highly ritualised, often enveloped in a series of narratives and rites. In South Africa, this is particularly visible among the Xhosa community where boys are sent to "the mountain" to live off the land and learn basic principles around being "real" men.

This rite and the implications it has for the HIV epidemic constituted the core of Tshemese's research. By spending time in the bush in the Eastern Cape during initiation season, he was able to produce journalism that offers a first-hand account of the ritual, at the same time exposing the malpractice, myths and HIV risks that have come to mar the traditional procedure.

Having been privy to some of the exchanges between the initiates, in "Testing the Mercedes", Tshemese can share the sexually risky myth that initiates have to "try out" and "cleanse" their newly circumcised penises by sleeping with someone they consider of lesser value first. By recounting the initiates' misguided bravado, and contrasting it with the views of experts, the article reveals the practice's vulnerability to charlatan traditional surgeons and attendants who have come to severely erode the value of initiations.

Malpractice within TMC takes a high toll every year, with deaths and botched procedures receiving a considerable amount of media coverage. Thus, in highlighting this, Tshemese opted for a more narrative angle in "A woman who saves lives", where he tells the story of a female doctor who has advocated tirelessly for safer practices. Her experience also suggests that there may be hope for reconciling the medical practice with the traditional rite.

On the whole, growing awareness of TMC's volatility has helped galvanise some government intervention. Tshemese's series also takes this into consideration, but his in-depth research allows him to tell the story through the eyes of the men whom the health department employs as custodians. Thus, "A day in the lives of the guardians" starts off as a personal narrative, but as the backdrop against which these interactions play off becomes increasingly apparent, the focus shifts to expose a context that informs risky traditional circumcisions and poor aftercare.

Outside Xhosa culture, circumcision has not been widely practised in South Africa.[1] However, during the course of Tshemese's research in 2009, MMC gained considerable clout as an HIV-prevention method. In 2007, evidence from three trails culminated in the acceptance by the WHO and UNAIDS of MMC as a viable

---

1   A 2010 WHO report estimates that 35 per cent of the adult male population is circumcised (WHO and UNAIDS, 2010). The Zulu community abandoned circumcision under the rule of King Shaka Zulu around the turn of the eighteenth century, though there is talk of reinstituting this practice following the incumbent, King Goodwill Zwelithini's, open support for medical male circumcision (IRIN, 2009).

means of HIV prevention.[2] The trials showed that a circumcised man is 60 per cent less likely to contract HIV during vaginal sex than his uncircumcised peers.[3] While HIV had previously entered the fray in discussions around the safety of traditional circumcisions, this new evidence turned the tables – transforming circumcision from a potential "HIV threat" to a possible "HIV solution".[4]

Prior to the introduction of this new evidence, a number of physiological arguments already existed for the removal of the foreskin, including significantly reduced probability of penile cancer, genital ulcer disease, human papillomavirus (HPV) and a host of STIs (specifically syphilis) as well as decreased likelihood of urinary tract infection. For women, a circumcised partner means reduced risk of cervical cancer as well as chlamydia, bacterial vaginosis and trichomas.[5] But in South Africa it was the severity of the HIV epidemic that would convince government to introduce the service to public health facilities.[6] As a result, the 2007–2011 National Strategic Plan on HIV, STIs and TB flagged circumcision as a potential policy issue deserving further investigation.[7]

Thus, when Wilson Johwa commenced his fellowship with the project in 2010, the commotion surrounding MMC made it an obvious choice for more in-depth journalism. During the course of his tenure with the project, the Department of Health increasingly backed the large-scale rollout of MMC. So called "chop shops" were

2   WHO and UNAIDS (2007).

3   Auvert, Taljaard, Lagarde, Sobngwi-Tambekou, Sitta and Puren (2005).

4   See, for instance, Vincent (2008).

5   Morris and Castellsague (2011).

6   That the procedure had already been piloted successfully locally (Orange Farm was one of the three clinical trial sites), further bolstered the case for large-scale circumcision.

7   SANAC (2006).

set up in heavily affected areas and communication campaigns were launched. The message was clear: Men, step up and take charge of your sexual health. This included concerted efforts at dovetailing MMC with a more comprehensive safe-sex approach to ensure men continue to condomise and avoid high-risk behaviour, such as engaging in multiple partnerships.

Johwa's research tracks the introduction of MMC to South Africa's HIV-prevention package, unpacking the science that backs it, debunking misconceptions and following the progress of government's proposed rollout. Johwa's journalism makes it clear that properly integrating MMC into the country's HIV-prevention package – already comprising a range of medical and behavioural interventions – is no small feat. Particularly, it required sensitivity towards existing traditional practices, and demands careful negotiation of concerns levelled by communication experts that not advising men that the procedure only offers partial HIV protection could undermine HIV efforts.

Johwa navigates this terrain skilfully by producing engaging yet highly informative journalism. This includes two blogs offering a behind-the-scenes view of the research, which were subsequently posted on the journAIDS website. Two of Johwa's articles were published in the first edition of *The New Age*. Three of Tshemese's four articles were printed in the *Saturday Dispatch*, the weekend edition of the *Daily Dispatch*, the Eastern Cape's most widely read publication. As initiation rituals are endemic to the region, TMC is a particular topic of interest for *Dispatch* readers.

A call to action

By 2012, over 250 000 MMC procedures had already been performed.[8] Late in 2011, the drive to circumcise was further vindicated. In Orange Farm, where a significant proportion of the population had been circumcised, the prevalence of HIV among circumcised men was found to be significantly lower than among their uncircumcised peers.[9] This "real world" evidence sealed the deal for MMC as a viable HIV-prevention method.

MMC is the first biomedical intervention in the HIV epidemic to be primarily targeted at heterosexual men. Previously, appeals had been almost entirely focused on behaviour. Often these would take on an admonishing tone: "Don't sleep around", "Don't have unprotected sex", "Don't be abusive." Now, rather than being reprimanded, men are called on to take action. Subsequently, images of men touted by MMC campaigns are of a "new" kind of man – sensitive, considerate, yet assertive and empowered. It may be too soon to say, but these new images of men could positively impact men's health-seeking behaviour.

For traditional leaders, specifically in communities where circumcision is already being practised traditionally, the rollout of MMC may pose some challenges and could take several years of advocacy to address.[10] In Orange Farm a kind of hybrid has been piloted where the medical procedure is incorporated into the traditional ritual. Boys are circumcised surgically but continue with the initiation ritual as usual.[11] This compromise does not only significantly lower the risk of contracting HIV during a traditional

---

8   SANAC (2011).

9   Auvert, Taljaard, Rech, Lissouba, Singh, Shabangu *et al.* (2011).

10   Crafford, A. "Cut and mistrust", *Mail & Guardian* (August 2009).

11   Taljaard, Shabangu, Mkhwanazi, Mashigo, Lissouba and Auvert (2010).

circumcision, but also ensures the initiates reap the full benefits of the procedure. This is particularly valid given growing evidence that many traditional procedures do not entail the full removal of the foreskin. Anecdotal evidence and some news coverage also suggests that much of the traditional procedure is already compromised by unethical practice, with some initiates openly lambasting the ritual, casting further doubt on the value of this practice.[12]

Does circumcision make the cut? Media images of traditional and medical male circumcision

In our period of analysis, coverage could be sectioned into two distinct camps: articles reporting on medical male circumcision; and those covering the traditional process.[13] This also played into how the coverage was distributed over time. While MMC made headlines at regular intervals, TMC coverage was largely isolated to the "circumcision season", which falls in the winter months (June–August).

Overall, a very distinct rift appears to characterise the local news media's coverage of circumcision, where the traditional ritual is treated as a separate entity to the medical procedure entirely. In our assessment, reports rarely made attempts to contrast or compare the two practices, and where there were calls for reconciling the two approaches, the motion was usually being put forward by either the medical camp or the sphere of academia.

---

12   Mgqolozana (2009).

13   Our year-long investigation ran from March 2011 to 2012. Using the keywords "medical male circumcision", and "circumcision" and running those through the HIV & AIDS Media Project's database, the search yielded 18 articles. For the keywords "traditional male circumcision", "traditional circumcision" and "initiation", the search brought up 16 articles. Additionally, newspapers were scanned by a trained researcher to include articles that related to the subjects that may have been omitted by the particular keywords.

Our analysis also revealed that, whereas the HIV benefit is often touted in MMC coverage, both HIV risk and benefit are glaringly absent from discussions around TMC. Furthermore, while the media are taking heed of circumcision and grant it a fair amount of airtime, coverage tends to be superficial and events-driven. Though some articles on the medical procedure and research backing it are fairly thorough, they often lack crucial context. As for what all of this may mean for ideas of being a man, reports were mostly silent.

Rituals gone wrong grab headlines

News coverage of traditional circumcision could again be broadly classified into four groups: reports of botched circumcision and malpractice; official response to malpractice; communities welcoming home initiates; and scandals associated with circumcision.

Most common in the TMC coverage were articles reporting malpractice by traditional attendants. As the gore in these stories make them very newsworthy, this is not particularly surprising. Regrettably, this kind of coverage does little more than pander to voyeurism. The articles in our analysis stopped short of asking pertinent questions about the management of initiation schools and instead tallied only deaths and quoted spokespeople's responses. None of the coverage mentioned the HIV risk posed by septic circumcisions and there was no mention of the protective benefit that MMC offers from HIV.

Second most common were stories of government action geared towards addressing risks in traditional procedures. This included a proposal to implement policy that would regulate traditional attendants, the dispatching of task teams to monitor the procedures and an official warning directed at communities to exercise caution when sending boys to initiation schools. Some of this coverage made links to sexual health but with varying degrees of sophistication.

All of the articles in this group failed to appropriate HIV risk to unregulated traditional practices, or to link to the health and HIV protection benefits offered by the medical procedure. Some, in fact, added more confusion. A *Daily Sun* article incorrectly framed the opening of a circumcision service in Soweto as a means to curb botched traditional circumcisions. The HIV-prevention benefits of circumcision – the primary reason for opening this site – go completely unmentioned.[14]

Another article quoted the Limpopo minister for local government, housing and traditional affairs saying that initiation schools are "entrusted by the government" to help curb sexually transmitted infections (STIs) and to teach men to lead "good lives".[15] The article does not elaborate on whether the spread of STIs would be curbed because of the biomedical rewards associated with the removal of the foreskin or whether this related more to the subsequent "good lives" comment. Only one report in the sample suggested that traditional procedures pose an HIV risk, but remained mum on the HIV benefits that MMC offers.[16]

A number of articles in the sample had a distinctly jovial tone, reporting on the return home of the initiates who had completed their rite of passage and were now officially "men". While this space offers an ideal opportunity to engage with what initiation means for masculinity, aside from one cursory mention that a particular school produces "responsible men", there was no further discussion on the subject.[17]

The final category comprised two articles that cover circum-

---

14   *Citizen* and SAPA. "New law may reduce botched circumcisions", *The Citizen* (August 2011).

15   Matlala, A. "Rules tightened for circumcision", *Sowetan* (June 2011).

16   Ngomane, E. "Warning against illegal circumcisions", *The Citizen* (June 2011).

17   Torerai, E. "Dithakong welcomes back its 90 initiates", *The New Age* (July 2011).

cision scandals. Notably, they were both from the popular tabloid *Daily Sun*, for which this kind of coverage is quite common. The first tells of the assault and involuntary circumcision of two old men by a group of boys, apparently themselves initiates.[18] The second article in the "scandal" camp reports the actions of a shady neighbour who sent the boy next door to an initiation camp without his parents' consent.[19] None of the articles mentions HIV risk or engages with the subject beyond merely listing events.

The remaining two articles in the study could be considered outliers. One column in *The New Age* investigates a costly government proposal to curb initiation deaths. This is couched in a wider discussion of how initiation relates to masculinity. The article also outlines circumcision benefits.[20] It is the only story in the sample that provided context and engaged meaningfully with the information.

The final article in our assessment presents a curious blend of science and superstition. It is a report in the *Daily Sun* on a ritual performed to cleanse a "cursed" initiation site. Apparently, the site had seen one fatal stabbing of an initiate by a traditional nurse, the murder of two gang members seeking refuge in one of the huts, as well as a fourth murder, which occurred during a brawl. While this hints strongly at poor management of the site, the community was in agreement that slaughtering a cow, goat and sheep would take care of the matter. This myth and superstition narrative is standard fare for the *Daily Sun*. Then a Western health narrative is introduced and the community's chief is quoted, saying they would like the authorities to train traditional attendants to use one blade per initiate and to start wearing gloves. Though the blend of traditional practice and science

---

18   Moobi, T. "Initiates cut madalas!", *Daily Sun* (June 2011).

19   Mkhondo, A. "Forced to go to initiation school", *Daily Sun* (June 2011).

20   Velhaphi, S. "Greed causes initiation deaths", *The New Age* (July 2011).

makes for an uneasy tone in the article, it does suggest there is scope for integrating medical procedures into TMC.

New cut sites make the news

In our assessment, coverage of medical male circumcision could be divided into three groups: articles dealing with proposed neonatal circumcision policy; coverage of the rollout of MMC services; and news items engaging with the science and research backing the procedure.

The first category relates to the debate that ensued when the Department of Health announced plans to include neonatal circumcision in its HIV-prevention strategy.[21] This coincided with the release of the first draft of the new National Strategic Plan in August 2011, within which these plans were contained.[22] The proposal was greeted with scepticism, particularly from local chiefs, who felt it would compromise the initiation ritual if boys were already circumcised as infants.[23] Also voicing concern were medical experts raising doubts around the HIV-prevention benefits offered by performing the procedure early in a boy's life.[24] The debate soon steered away from HIV entirely, as clamour ensued around fears that the cosmetic industry could exploit neonatal circumcision. As baby foreskins are a much sought-after ingredient in certain "miracle" cosmetics, experts from the Medical Rights Advocacy Group warned this could lead to illegal trade of foreskins.

---

21   This comprised a total of six articles within the 18 articles in total dealing with MMC that the study covered.

22   Govender, P. "Experts divided over baby circumcision plan", *Sunday Times* (August 2011).

23   Mwande, J. "Chiefs oppose infant 'snip'", *The New Age* (November 2011).

24   Govender, P. "Experts divided over baby circumcision plan", *Sunday Times* (August 2011).

The second category of MMC coverage tracked the rollout of adult medical male circumcision as part of government's MMC campaign. The coverage had an overall positive slant, often echoing government sentiment and encouraging men to circumcise. Two of the news items made mention of traditional circumcision, indicating that the procedure already had some significance in South Africa, beyond the purely medical.[25,26] Of the rollout coverage, two articles mention that circumcision offers up to 60 per cent protection from HIV. A third makes a more vague reference, stating only that circumcision has been "scientifically shown to reduce the risk of STIs and HIV".[27] None of the three stories mentioned that circumcision does not preclude condom use.

Among this sample was a promo-style article in the *Daily Sun* that reads: "MEN! Go and join the thousands of other men and get circumcised in order to slow HIV infection."[28] It is a direct appeal, showcasing the services of the Khula Ndoda Centre at Chris Hani Baragwanath Hospital in Soweto. Whether this is paid-for advertising is unclear as the article is set in the normal editorial fashion among other news pieces, its only distinguishing feature a grey box.

One article in this category covers the ANC Youth League's controversial call for compulsory circumcision. It quotes a South African Medical Association spokesperson stating that circumcision "reduces chances of HIV infection by 80 per cent".[29] This is patently false and rather alarmingly oversells the efficacy of the procedure.

The final article in the sample is taken from the *Daily Sun* and

25 Masinga, S. "Massive push for safe male circumcision", *The Star* (June 2011).

26 Mapumule, Z. "Male circumcision project progresses at limp pace", *The New Age* (March 2011).

27 Masinga, S. "Massive push for safe male circumcision", *The Star* (June 2011).

28 Ngcobo, N. "Circumcision helps fight HIV", *Daily Sun* (February 2012).

29 Moloto, M. "Call for compulsory circumcision", *The Star* (June 2011).

covers the opening of a new MMC site at Zola Clinic, Soweto. The article implies that MMC is a popular procedure, stating that over 200 procedures are completed daily at the clinic.[30] The local Minister for health is quoted, saying "all responsible people should grab such opportunities with both hands". But the article stays mum on the exact benefits of circumcision, missing an ideal opportunity to inform over four million readers.

The third major group of articles in our study engaged less with the rollout of MMC and more with its science. In one of the five articles in this group, circumcision forms part of a wider discussion around medical breakthroughs in the HIV response and is thus afforded relatively little airtime.[31] A second article deals with MMC in the context of debunking a series of HIV myths, specifying that circumcision does not "prevent" HIV infection, only "decreases the likelihood" of HIV infection and then goes on to explain why – because the foreskin contains cells much more susceptible to infection.[32] The remaining three articles have made MMC their central concern and engage quite extensively with the issue.

Our search yielded two more articles relating to MMC that could not be appropriated to any particular category. One, a column in the *Mail & Guardian*, is a zealous outcry at MMC efforts that challenges the science supporting the effectiveness of the procedure.[33] The second is a promotional insert in the *Daily Sun*, flighted as part of the Brothers for Life campaign, which in simple, clear language outlines the benefits of the procedure.[34]

---

30 Nkhwashu, G. "New cut site in Zola!", *Daily Sun* (August 2011).

31 Keeton, C. "Prevention breakthrough to boost Aids indaba", *Sunday Times* (June 2011).

32 Malan, M. "Exploding seven myths about HIV", *Mail & Guardian* (August 2011).

33 Barker, W. "Going off half-cocked – again", *Mail & Guardian* (July 2011).

34 "Look after your health and your sex life", *Daily Sun* (July 2011).

Our analysis and the journalism showcased here suggest that there is still much ground to be covered in hashing out the intricacies that characterise the national conversation around circumcision. Particularly, much work remains to be done in reconciling the traditional rite with the medical, more HIV-prevention-focused approach. While the media have been following these developments, very few of the tough questions have been sufficiently interrogated. There also remains a marked need to emphasise the protective benefit of the procedure while advocating for the use of additional protective measures, such as condoms.

References /

Auvert, B; Taljaard, D; Lagarde, E; Sobngwi-Tambekou, J; Sitta, R; and Puren, A. (2005) "Randomized, controlled intervention trial of male circumcision for reduction of HIV infection risk: the ANRS-1265 trial." *PLoS Medicine*, 2(298).

Auvert, B; Taljaard, D; Rech, D; Lissouba, P; Singh, B; Shabangu, D. *et al.* (2011) *Effect of the Orange Farm (South Africa) male circumcision roll-out (ANRS-12126) on the spread of HIV*. Abstract presented at the 6th IAS Conference on HIV Pathogenisis, Prevention and Treatment. Retrieved 4 April 2012, http://pag.ias2011.org/Abstracts.aspx?SID=43&AID=4792.

Hankins, C. (2007) "Male circumcision: Implications for women as sexual partners and parents." *Reproductive Health Matters*, 15(29).

IRIN. "Zulu king revives male circumcision." (15 December 2009) Retrieved 5 May 2012, http://www.irinnews.org/Report/87441/SOUTH-AFRICA-Zulu-king-revives-male-circumcision.

Mgqolozana, T. (2009) *A man who is not a man*. Pietermaritzburg: University of KwaZulu-Natal Press.

Morris, BJ and Castellsague, X. (2011) "The role of circumcision in preventing STIs." *Sexually Transmitted Infections and Sexually Transmitted Diseases*, 54.

SANAC. (2006) *HIV & AIDS and STI Strategic Plan for South Africa, 2007–2011*. South African National AIDS Council, Department of Health.

SANAC. (2011) *National Strategic Plan on HIV, STIs and TB, 2012–2016*. South African National AIDS Council, Department of Health.

Taljaard, D; Shabangu, D; Mkhwanazi, A; Mashigo, T; Lissouba, P; and Auvert, B. (2010) *Traditional initiation and medical male circumcision collaborating: going to the medical mountain?* Poster presented at the 18th International AIDS Conference, Vienna, Austria. Retrieved 4 April 2012, http://pag.aids2010.org/Abstracts.aspx?AID=6186.

Vincent, L. (2008) "'Boys will be boys': Traditional Xhosa male circumcision, HIV and sexual socialisation in contemporary South Africa." *Culture, Health & Sexuality*, 10(5).

WHO and UNAIDS. (2010) "Progress in male circumcision scale-up: country implementation and research update." June 2010.

WHO and UNAIDS. (2007) *Male circumcision: Global trends and determinants of prevalence, safety and acceptability*. Geneva.

Separating the boys from the men / Journalism

Testing the Mercedes

Mthetho Tshemese

Sathan'udanile uThix'uvumile singaw'amadoda halala, halala halala halala. "Satan is disappointed and God is great and has made us men, hooray hooray hooray."

On the Mount Ruth Station road between East London and King William's Town, a beautiful melody reverberates. *Abakweta* (initiates) are singing and dancing, ululating and whistling, to the amusement of motorists, who honk their horns.

It is a sunny winter's morning in 2009 – a time of celebration for these young men, who just spent a month in *Sacramento*, a nickname given to their initiation site. It was time for 18 of the 40 initiates to go home the following day. They would no longer be *amakhwenkwe* (boys) or *abakwetha* but *amadoda* (men). They had completed the traditional initiation course and now had status in society as men. The singing initiates were on their way to the Buffalo River to wash, in preparation for their trip back into the township. There, celebratory ceremonies had already started.

Describing his elation, Mawonga, 18, says his main excitement is to check if sex would be the same as when he still had the "poloneck". His companions giggle. "So, my friend, you want to test your Mercedes Benz [penis] and iron it?" asks Thando, 17.

Ntobeko, who looks 14 but claims to be 17, says every initiated man knows he should test and iron his Mercedes Benz. His peers nod in agreement and Vuyani, 17, adds that anyone who claimed he didn't was ignorant or had never been initiated.

Asked why their penises were Mercedes Benzes, rather than Toyotas or Nissans, they burst into laughter. Zola, 18, lifts his blanket and addresses his newly healed penis: "Gees, my brother, they say you are a Toyota. Never!"

Mdantsane township is the second largest township in South Africa. Situated 20 kilometres west of East London, it has an urban pulse and feel, yet its residents are deeply rooted in their Xhosa cultural and traditional rituals.

Despite attempts to curb botched circumcisions, a number of initiates still die, while others end up in hospital. Yet, during winter and summer holidays, many boys continue to go to the initiation schools.

Mbulelo Dyasi, coordinator of Men's Projects at the Masimanyane Women's Support Centre, believes the initiation process "has no order and is a haven for drug activities and promotes gender violence against women and girl children".

Set up in 1995 in East London, the non-profit organisation focuses on gender-based violence, sexual and reproductive health, and the gendered nature of HIV and AIDS. In his office, Dyasi holds an unpublished report about the teachings taking place at some initiation schools. The information it contains is alarming.

"Look, when you challenge these things, your masculinity is doubted and questioned. I do not care if iNkosi [Chiefs] deny what is happening at these initiation schools. The reality is that there are a lot of bad things being taught to young boys at these initiation schools and in fact a lot of them are nothing but gangsterism initiation schools."

Fixing his spectacles, he adds: "You can say I am being harsh, but that is the reality for many schools here in the Eastern Cape. Around

2006, there were newspaper reports about graduate initiates raping women, including the elderly."

Incidents like this were reported in Zwelitsha, greater King William's Town, Engcobo, and other areas. In 2006, a 27-year-old woman was gang-raped by nine graduate initiates. "I mean, if we are supposed to teach these boys to be men, then how come they come from the initiation schools and do these horrible things?"

His Masimanyane colleagues agree. One adds: "I can see that you are shocked, but let me ask you something. What is the profile of *amakhankatha* [traditional nurses] who look after the initiates? Actually, these people are supposed to teach the initiates about being a man and yet, if you go to the initiation schools, you find a lot of unemployed, homeless, illiterate and ignorant people.

"Even worse, you find people with criminal records being part of the people teaching these initiates about manhood. When these boys come out of the initiation schools, they have a different language, which is supposedly deep isiXhosa but in fact it is gang language and appropriated from the number gang language from prison. They call it *Shalambombo*."

In 2009, the Masimanyane organisation held three youth summits in East London, Engcobo and King William's Town.

The young men spoke of pressure to have sex to "cleanse themselves". They were told to avoid sleeping with loved ones because they would give them bad luck. Instead, they were encouraged to sleep with someone they did not love. Young women who attended the summit said they were reluctant to sleep with graduated initiates, for fear of having bad luck deposited in them.

The main reason for having sex immediately after initiation is to test if the new Mercedes Benz works effectively. It is also through sex that they rid themselves of extreme bad luck. They believe they should *sula*, or wipe it off, by sleeping with someone of "lesser value" than a loved one. The longer they take to "get rid" of the dirt, the longer they carry it inside and the more their aspirations are frustrated.

Dyasi warns that, with low employment rates and lack of opportunities, young men believe they cannot afford the added burden of bad luck. This means women are more vulnerable to HIV since they are seen as "objects" into whom dirt can be deposited.

The young men believe they needed to "iron" their penises or they might never heal properly.

"Now, what kind of men are we developing in these schools and why must these boys think you still need to do things outside the initiation school to heal properly? I can tell you a lot of people are going to be angry about us questioning these things but, as Africans, we like defending nonsense.

"In Zwelitsha we once found out that *abakwetha* were having sex at the initiation school and [traditional nurses] had girlfriends with whom they slept during the course of the initiation process too.

"So, now we promote multiple and concurrent sexual partners because it is our culture and these boys must iron their penises? Yes, these things happen easily because many men do not go to the bush to check on the boys – not unless their children or nephews are there. Now who monitors what happens and what is taught in these initiation schools?"

According to the Soul City Institute for Health and Development Communication, multiple and concurrent sexual partnerships, with low consistent condom use, have been identified as key drivers of the HIV pandemic in southern Africa. In surveys, a sexual partnership is considered to be concurrent if a person reports having two or more sexual partners in a month. Other drivers have been shown to be male attitudes to sex and sexual behaviour, gender and sexual violence.

In his 2004 *(Un)real AIDS Review*, clinical psychologist Dr Kgamadi Kometsi looked at "dominant images of men" and found that initiates were encouraged to test themselves sexually after graduating from the initiation school. When Kometsi asked one of his respondents: "So you are encouraged to go and test yourself? Let's say when you go to *esuthwini* [initiation school], you are in a committed relationship. You have been involved for some time before you went. When you come back, where are you going to test yourself, on her?"

The respondent replied: "Not on her. There's a perception that when you come back from *esuthwini*, you are carrying dirt. So you have to deposit the dirt somewhere else. Otherwise if you test on your girlfriend, that relationship is not going to last."

Dyasi, who is also Primary Prevention Officer and Public Educator for Masimanyane, is animated about possible solutions. Leaning back in his chair, he laughs. "Yes, there are solutions but it is not going to be particular groups that will solve our problems. Everyone must do their job.

"The Health Department cannot be at the forefront of traditional circumcision but, because these boys go to hospitals, they have to do something. The Chiefs cannot do it alone also because some parents dump their own kids in the bush with [traditional nurses] they don't even know very well. Maybe families should hold interviews before appointing traditional nurses and they must check their health knowledge and other skills, such as counselling, but also check if he has a criminal record or not.

"I am happy that Chiefs are busy working on a curriculum to be taught in these initiation schools and I hope there will be content on human rights, sex and gender, and that there will be an improvement on the profiling of the traditional nurses so that we reduce criminality and gangsterism in the bush."

Originally published as "Gangsterism in the bush" in the Saturday Dispatch *on 26 June 2010.*

A day in the lives of the guardians

Mthetho Tshemese

To curb the high incidence of botched circumcisions, the Depart-
ment of Health in the Eastern Cape has appointed Designated
Medical Officers to supervise traditional initiations and expose
misconduct. Mthetho Tshemese spends time with the men who see
to it that the boys of their communities are ushered into manhood
without incident.

Breakfast consisted of carrots, peas, rice with beef curry, grilled
bacon, rolls, chicken giblets and two litres of Sparletta – *Pine Nut*
flavour. Yesterday it was boiled ox head with steamed bread.

Breathing heavily, Bra Munda explains: "This food is the aphrodi-
siac that keeps you erect and ready. Let us go, gentlemen, we are late
and the initiates are dying while we are here eating."

Every winter and summer holidays thousands of young boys go
through traditional male circumcision and are initiated from boyhood to manhood in the Eastern Cape and other parts of the country.
The initiation process is the embodiment of amaXhosa masculinity.

Since 2001, when a law was introduced to make these circumcisions safer, the Health MEC selects health practitioners to conduct
medical examinations, register traditional surgeons and nurses and
conduct initiation site visits. By means of these "bush trackings",
Bra Munda and his colleagues, Bra H, Zizi and Madiba, can monitor initiation schools and initiates' progress. These four Designated
Medical Officers (DMOs) are based at Cecilia Makiwane Hospital in
Mdantsane township, East London.

For the 2009 winter season, there were over 400 *abakwetha*
(initiates) in Mdantsane and surrounding areas. Only 100 of these

were 18 years or older – the legal age for circumcision. The majority, spurred on by peer pressure, were just 16.

Fatalities keep the Eastern Cape in the spotlight. Despite the Application of Health Standards in Traditional Circumcision Act, the 2009 winter season saw 54 deaths and many more botched circumcisions.

The 2001 Act makes it a criminal offence to run an illegal school or circumcise a child without parental consent. Every initiate must receive a pre-circumcision medical certificate from a medical officer.

A DMO since 2004, Bra H notes: "Circumcision is very complicated and has always been. There were people before us ... who used to deal with circumcision like we are, but it seems it is getting more complicated."

Earlier that morning, the DMOs received a phone call reporting alleged negligence in Ncerha, a rural village between East London and Port Alfred. As the group prepares to leave, both Bra Munda and Bra H are on their cellphones verifying information.

"You see, the case we are attending to now is of a registered *ikhankatha* [traditional nurse]. But the allegation against him suggests he is operating like an illegal one," Bra Munda explains. "He is accused of leaving an initiate unattended for five days. I mean, how do you do that and what is the point of being a registered nurse if you become grossly negligent?"

It is often towards the end of the circumcision period, just when they thought the boys were going home, that complications are reported. Many of the calls received by the DMOs are from women – even though women are not permitted to go to the bush and generally don't see the boys. Bra H explains that women often get their information from the young boys who bring food to the initiation schools. They become concerned by reports of an initiate's poor appetite, his disturbed sleeping patterns or being left alone in the hut with no men around.

"Nowadays, you even have cellular phones and I would not be surprised if some of the *abakwetha* talk to their mothers or even send pictures to them while they are at the initiation school.

"A lot of men have this idea that we should inflict pain in the bush and that, when an initiate complains of pain or discomfort, he is being a sissy. So in most cases, men who are in the bush and see *umkwetha* complaining will say this is what is expected here, and there is no crisis at all."

So much demand was placed on the DMOs during the initiation season, they say they struggled to cope. "We are not the holy spirit," says Bra Munda. "We can't be everywhere at once. People must take responsibility for their children ... Now they are calling us, but we are just medical officers. Where are the men in these communities, where is the leadership? I mean if someone neglects *umkwetha*, that person is known to the community. Now we must drive there from Mdantsane. Are we going to sort that problem out better than the community can?"

Bra H laughs as Bra Munda continues. "You know what? During pre-circumcision we do health talks and even teach would-be initiates about different illnesses and how to identify and manage them during initiation ... Some of them even disclose their HIV-positive status to us and we counsel them. But the minute they are in the bush, I think families, especially men and the community structures, should monitor *abakwetha*. Most of them don't even bother visiting their own children. By the time they go to the bush the initiate has a serious complication."

No longer laughing, Bra H leans forward, and adds: "In reality, a complication does not become major overnight. If people went regularly to the initiation sites ... and took responsibility for their children, they would pick up complications very early. Most of the time, they behave as though it is our primary duty to look after their children – and it's theirs really."

During the drive, the conversation moves back to the importance of eating for potency. The mood lightens as the men discuss sex, erectile dysfunction, and the need for men to satisfy women. But before long, the talk returns to some of the men's young charges who were forced to have their penises amputated. Others would never manage an erection again. All were left with deep emotional scars and still have to deal with rejection from their communities.

Bra H leans back and looks out of the window. "Our job is very painful and what hurts the most is that a lot of people think it is us who should do more. Yet they are the ones who should prepare their children and monitor their progress in the bush.

"There are many good traditional nurses, but some of them are not, even though they are registered with us. It is not for us to make that call when people send and risk their children to bad characters."

There is silence as the car approaches Village 7 in Ncerha. The second car, driven by Madiba, is marked with a Department of Health logo. Villagers respond with curiosity.

The initiate's father refuses to get into the car, but prefers to walk to the *ibhoma* hut, where *umkwetha* are staying. The DMOs explain that most people don't want to be seen in a health department car while their child is an *umkwetha*. Anything that would start gossip is avoided as it could bring stigma to the child and his family.

The DMOs park on the main road and walk past a livestock feeding camp. As they approach, three faces, white with clay, can be seen chatting to the father. A 71-year-old local elder, known by his clan name Ngqothoza Rhadebe, is incensed. Waving his knobkierie, he yells: "As far as I am concerned, my son, I want to *moer* this traditional nurse and he must tell us, where did he ever see the act of leaving an initiate unattended for five days?"

After inspecting the three initiates, the DMOs are happy. Two are ready to go home. The third, though not satisfactory, is also not critical. The DMOs treat him and make recommendations. A fourth initiate had apparently run away. Circumcised illegally, he was afraid of being arrested. Bra Munda says this is common. An initiate would attend initiation school illegally and run away every time they conduct bush trackings.

The elder reported that he was one of very few men who visited initiation schools in Ncerha. He wasn't sure if anyone taught young men about masculinity at these schools.

As the DMOs prepared to leave, the initiates asked who would teach them *izipatula,* the new men's language. If no one did, how would they authenticate themselves as "real" men? Their faces reflected their anxiety.

They had every reason to be worried. It is common for communities to call gatherings of *amakrwala,* to check for the "real" men versus those suspected of having gone to hospital or used Western medicine. These young men are referred to by the derogatory terms *ilulwane* or *unotywetywe.* Such gatherings can become violent and have sometimes led to deaths.

The DMOs try to reassure the initiates. What matters is that they have gone through the ritual. Now they needed to conduct themselves accordingly and be better men. They should be responsible citizens who find solutions to their community problems.

But these initiates would still have to face suspicion from other *amakrwala* about the legitimacy and authenticity of their masculinity. The DMOs say their greatest challenge is that the teachings at initiation schools are not always consistent with what they would like to see them be taught.

"This thing [checking who are the real men] is the same as the teachings that some boys receive, to sleep around to assert their virility and masculinity; the drugs they take here, the stolen property that gets hidden here. But at the end of the day it is not only our job to monitor initiates. Communities and families must take responsibility for what their children are taught."

The DMOs have called on members of the Ncerha community, including a community leader. He promised to hold a meeting, to mobilise the community to take responsibility for their initiates and hold the traditional nurse accountable. Later, the DMOs report that the community of Ncerha formed a circumcision committee that would oversee all circumcision-related matters. They would in future have three traditional nurses.

The initiate who ran away was later found.

Makers of men

Mthetho Tshemese

*"They go because they want to confirm that indeed they are men
... dying to be a man is better than living with a fragile and uncertain masculine identity."*

Andile Qwanyisa watches as a silver-grey Opel Astra pulls up. "Wait
– this is shocking ..." he says. Covered in white clay and carrying a
knobkierie, the driver gets out. The second occupant takes his place
in the driver's seat and, as the car drives away, Andile remarks: "That
one is not mine. Where have you seen an initiate driving a car?"

Andile (49) is a respected and experienced *ikhankatha*, a traditional attendant or nurse, who cares for boys during the traditional
initiation ritual. Required by law to be registered, traditional attendants' primary role is to treat the circumcision wound and manage
the physical and emotional health of initiates. They are also supposed
to teach life skills and prepare them for life as men, with discipline
and respect being central to their "curriculum".

Kuwait, an initiation site, is situated in a semirural area near
Mdantsane township. The site has 40 initiation huts and is run by
Andile. Kuwait was given its name in the 1980s because "it is not a
place for quitters".

Andile has been a traditional attendant since 1986 – a mere six
years after he was an initiate himself. He looks after an average of 35
initiates every season, in winter and summer. He learned his trade
from the best attendant in the area and has never had a single death
or hospitalisation.

Two community members, who have come to visit their sons,
attest to this. Ngakum Joji (72), says: "We hear things from the radio

and watch on TV where shocking things happen. I swear on my mother we have never had those here and all our children go through those tiny hands of this young man [pointing at Andile]. Don't underestimate them because they are tiny, for they do a great job."

Sandile Mabala (57) has come to visit his son and nephew, who are initiates under Andile's care. "Another thing is that Andile knows that there are people who come here frequently. We tell him when we are not happy about something and he is receptive to criticism."

Mabala wishes Andile could teach attendants in places where initiates are dying or being hospitalised. Covering his mouth with his hand, Andile smiles and shakes his head: "I am just doing my job and don't want to talk about other people's jobs because then I will be accused of thinking that I am clever."

And yet Andile is not happy about some of the men he has produced. "Our job is to make boys heal. But some of them go out to do horrible things. Some rob people, some are in jail, and some rape."

Thando *"Tbo"* (Touch) Mfenyana is Andile's assistant. The 22-year-old Touch, like many of his peers, calls his mentor "Sir Ands", after Sir Alex Fergusson of Manchester United. Andile likens Touch to a soccer player who has potential to be a star, but still plays for the development team. "One day I will promote him … For now he must watch and learn and carry the lamp while I work. When I want to sleep I ask him to look after the initiates and he is showing promise."

About 10 kilometres west of Kuwait is Rwanda. It is headed by Mzukisi Siyo aka Magali, who is also a traditional surgeon, with two assistants. At present, all three are struggling to come to terms with the death of an initiate just days before.

"Do you know that, here in Rwanda, it was for the first time ever to have an initiate dying?" asks Sakhumzi, one of Magali's assistants, who speaks passionately about their work. Magali is quick to point out the boy's attendant was not registered, nor was he known to them, but was chosen by the initiate's family. He believes that families should come to them, as the main attendants, to verify an attendant's credentials before entrusting them to look after their children.

Even though he heads Rwanda, Magali reports that he could not interfere with the other attendants' work as he was brought in by the boy's family. Magali and his team find it difficult to accept the death.

Unathi, who has been sitting quietly, now pipes up: "The negligent attendant must be arrested even though that is not going to reverse the death of that initiate. But the initiate's family are the ones who will decide on laying charges against him. Personally, I don't want to ever see him here in Rwanda."

Magali says, in Rwanda, they focus on doing their job well. But he is concerned their reputation is under threat because of the negligence of others.

The site was originally called Barcelona. But in 1995, during a very hot season, the attendants saw fire and thought the initiates were going home, because the huts are usually burnt when initiates graduate from the school.

"In actual fact it was an accident at one hut that caused the fire, but the flames quickly spread to other huts," Sakhumzi explains. "There was chaos, with everyone running and screaming. Since then we called the place Rwanda as it reminded us of the time when people of Rwanda did not have a place to run to. For us we felt like we were in Rwanda and this place is still called Rwanda even today."

The names of both camps are deeply significant, according to Malose Langa, a Wits Psychology lecturer and PhD candidate conducting research on masculinity: "The choice of names for the sites is fascinating and could be telling us about the life and death dynamic that has become part of the initiation process. These young men know that during every initiation season there will be boys who will die and some will get hospitalised and some may even lose their penises … Yet they go because they want to confirm that indeed they are men. The unconscious driver could be that dying to be a man is better than living with a fragile and uncertain masculine identity."

Langa says many men become involved in risky activities – such as illegal car racing, train surfing and gang wars. Others have sex with multiple and concurrent partners. "These activities somehow confirm to them and the world that they are men."

Masculinity is a fragile identity, the existence of which needs to be confirmed, maintained and performed to feed the psyche of a man. Langa suggests that "we need to change the script of what a man is and find healthier narratives of what makes one a man".

For Eastern Cape Xhosa boys, the only way to become *indoda,* a man, is by going through the traditional circumcision and initiation into manhood. Once you acquire this status, you become a respected member of society with an acceptable and desirable masculine identity.

In contrast, *inkwenkwe,* a boy, has neither honour nor respect, as is clear from the Xhosa phrase: *Inkwenkwe yinja,* a boy is a dog. It is not uncommon for teenage girls to say dismissively, "I don't date 'boys'", referring to anyone who has not been circumcised.

Unosala, a term used for a boy whose peers have gone for initiation, is as undesirable as being referred to as a dog. Teenage boys end up enduring immense pressure to become men and at times this leads to their being circumcised too early and illegally.

With both Rwanda and Kuwait having impressive records of wound management, Andile points out that being a man is more than just the removal of one's foreskin: "I tell my initiates that if they do wrong things, it does not matter if they went through initiation. If they do bad things afterwards, to me you are not *indoda,* a real man, but *indodi,* a fake man."

Originally published as "Risking life to be a man" in the Saturday Dispatch *on 3 July 2010.*

A woman who saves lives

Mthetho Tshemese

Traditional male circumcision is an area usually barred to women. But when she saw the extent to which botched procedures were affecting the boys in her community, this doctor couldn't help but get involved.

Dr Elizabeth Mamisa Chabula Nxiweni remembers when she was called to treat two boys from Peddie, a village between King William's Town and Grahamstown, who had just gone through their traditional circumcision ritual. One was 18, the other 20. She found the boys lying on their backs, both hands behind their heads, looking up at the ceiling. The room was silent.

"When I examined them, these kids had stumps – no penises at all. The elders from Peddie somehow had hoped that their penises would regenerate. But the initiates knew that this was not going to be the case. One of the boys asked me. 'Mama, what have we done to deserve this?'"

She removes her glasses and rubs her eyes. Dr Chabula Nxiweni is a 62-year-old Port Elizabeth medical doctor who has been involved in traditional male circumcision more than any other woman in the Eastern Cape – or South Africa for that matter.

Born in Korsten, she is the only girl of 10 children. She has 10 children of her own, five boys and five girls. Her eldest child is 40 and the youngest is 23.

Taking a deep breath, she tells of another three boys she treated after they were hospitalised. "One of these boys had gangrene and was rotten. As medical people, we have to remove rot. This boy from Dubu needed radical surgery and, after seeing him, I was ding-dong emotionally.

"I went to the second initiate. He was just 18 years old and his expression was different from that of other boys. I asked him: 'What is wrong, my child?' He looked away, lifted his sheet and said: '*Jonga, Mama.*' Look, Mama … That was one of the most difficult and painful pictures of my entire medical career."

Dr Chabula Nxiweni became involved in male circumcision in 1988 – an area traditionally barred to women, even medical doctors. A group of men brought four initiates, dressed in overalls, to see her in Motherwell.

"It was broad daylight and I tried to refer the old men to male doctors. I was already worried about the stigma associated with initiates who come to see a doctor, let alone a female doctor. Trying to protect the young men's reputations, I asked the old men to bring the initiates at 10 in the evening."

Once she had examined them at her surgery, she found herself in foreign territory. "These kids had all kinds of things which were foreign to me covering their wounds. And some were dehydrated and looked emotionally drained."

She called on her younger brother, Bra Deyi, to help her manage the initiates' wounds, while she focused on her role as medical doctor.

"Traditional circumcision is foreign territory for the Xhosa woman and there was no way I could have been able to handle everything without having someone, a man, to assist me. Besides, I could not go to the bush or even treat children publicly because of the stigma in the township when boys go to hospital or use Western medicine."

In June 1989, Dr Chabula Nxiweni saw another six initiates, one of whom had to be hospitalised. In December she was brought another 10. She was shocked that three groups of initiates had cigarette burns on their thighs.

"The initiates must have complained about pain, were told to stick it out and then got punished for being weak."

At this stage, she approached the Motherwell Community Development Forum to seek a mandate to address the traditional surgeons and nurses. She told them "children are dying and some have septic circumcisions".

Bra Deyi, who accompanied her, said: "Fathers, there is a problem, children are dying."

Every Sunday afternoon during 1990, she was invited to meetings of the traditional surgeons and nurses. Yet they would never agree that there was a problem. She saw more initiates during June and December of that year.

She believes the men of Port Elizabeth were uncertain about her bona fides. They found it difficult to relate to a woman who was interested in traditional male circumcision – it had never happened before. So it was only in 1991 that there was a breakthrough, when the traditional surgeons and nurses acknowledged that, indeed, there was a problem. Maybe they had been watching her to see if she was sincere, or just wanted to make money from the ritual.

"I asked them to map the way forward and they suggested establishing the Motherwell Traditional Surgeons and Attendants Association. This was exciting to me because it was out of their own accord that they formed this association and they designed their own code of conduct ... They raised issues that they wanted to tackle, which included inconsistent prices, traditional practitioners who got drunk at work, dealing with medical conditions such as HIV and other STIs, TB, diabetes, heart diseases, epilepsy."

Through the Association's interventions, "One boy, One blade" was adopted as a slogan. This was a significant achievement in minimising HIV risk and other infections among initiates. The Association also developed a comprehensive pre-circumcision medical examination form.

With a broad smile, Dr Chabula Nxiweni points out: "You know what? Pre-circumcision medical check-ups started in Motherwell in

1991 ... People might think that, as a woman, I was just forward and had nothing to do with traditional circumcision. Some men in this province used to come to my surgery at night and seek help because they were too scared to acknowledge that they had problems which, as men, they had caused and needed assistance."

Commenting on continued initiate deaths, Dr Chabula Nxiweni says the first step is for everyone to accept that there is a problem. "In Motherwell we acknowledged there was a problem and for years now we don't have deaths in Motherwell. And the men are driving the process forward."

When the government introduced legislation in 2001 to make traditional circumcision safer, Dr Chabula Nxiweni withdrew her involvement. Yet, despite all that she has seen, she still believes in traditional circumcision and talks passionately about the African philosophy that underpins it.

She recalls Zuko (not his real name), who was fitted with a prosthesis after losing his penis. She asked him how he felt about traditional circumcision. He replied that it was still relevant, but the initiates had to be looked after very well. If he had children, he would even send them to initiation school.

"Now that should tell you something, if someone who was hurt by the ritual can say that. You know I read an article in one of the papers by Andile Mngxitama who says traditional circumcision must be abolished. I feel sorry for him. I think he has a serious identity problem."

As a woman, of course, Dr Chabula Nxiweni has been dismissed for never having been through the ritual herself. "Yes, it is true. I am a woman and am not circumcised, but the difference is that I dedicated myself and worked with people who are knowledgeable ... and tried to find solutions. In Motherwell, since 1994, we have not had deaths of initiates. It is easier to sit and condemn and say abolish it, as if everything about traditional male circumcision is bad."

Dr Chabula Nxiweni feels the greatest problem in traditional circumcision is wound management and poverty. She also worries about the monitoring of traditional nurses.

"The ritual teaches initiates about restraint. Not everything you see you must touch or take. That is why, back in the day, you had to stay for months without having sex or eating certain foods before you went to the mountain. Our forefathers knew that a sexually transmitted illness would not show up immediately ... hence, you had to restrain yourself before going for initiation. Also, our traditions are against abuse of women and that is why you would hear: 'When you are angry, humble yourself and take a walk to cool off. Violence does not build family households.'"

But now she asks if these lessons are taught during initiation and who is doing the teaching? Years ago, she suggested having a circumcision village with a lecture hall, where young men would be taught to be good men for their families and communities.

If people knew what was intended by this ritual, Dr Chabula Nxiweni feels society would not have many of the problems it does. Men would not rape women and children and men would protect their wives from HIV and other illnesses. Parents would know that parental supervision was non-negotiable, especially for initiates.

"If we were sincere about our efforts to curb the deaths of initiates, there should have been a delegation of good traditional surgeons and traditional attendants being sent to the Pondoland long ago. As I said, *mntanam* [my child], this is too politicised now and there are many 'experts' whose intentions ..." she trails off. "I doubt whether they are noble and sincere."

Originally published as "A woman who saves initiates" in the Saturday Dispatch *on 24 July 2010.*

Bulking up HIV prevention

Wilson Johwa

In South Africa, where only 35 per cent of men are circumcised,
a scale-up of voluntary medical male circumcision will give men
the option to choose whether to undergo the procedure that offers
protection against HIV.

Voluntary medical male circumcision is due to be stepped up, with the government expecting provinces to take the lead in the roll-out. The proposed mass campaign follows acceptance in 2007 by the World Health Organization and the United Nations Joint Programme on HIV/AIDS (UNAIDS) that male circumcision provides 50 to 60 per cent protection against HIV for men.

"We regard it as the next frontier [in the fight against HIV] because it was not widely practised in our hospitals," says Health Minister Dr Aaron Motsoaledi, whose department has already produced a draft strategy.

KwaZulu-Natal has taken the lead with a target of 2.5 million voluntary medical male circumcisions by 2015. "The next province I'm speaking to is Mpumalanga because they also have a high [HIV] prevalence rate and eventually it will be all the provinces," explains Dr Motsoaledi.

KZN is the province worst affected, with an HIV prevalence of 25.8 per cent among both men and women in the 15–49 age group, followed by Mpumalanga with 23.1 per cent, while the lowest incidence of HIV (5.3 per cent) is in the Western Cape.

The national scale-up is proceeding as other countries in the region have already included medical male circumcision in their HIV-prevention packages. Swaziland's expansion started with "circumcision Saturdays" and is now targeting at least 150 000 men over the next five years. Botswana intends to circumcise 80 per cent of all males 0–49 years old by 2016.

However, male circumcision remains a contested procedure, both socially and medically.

The decision about whether to do it is also a very personal one. Jabu Khumalo (31), from Orlando West in Soweto, did it at Orange Farm to prevent premature ejaculation. "I just want the long strokes," he said.

Clinton Sebako (16) says: "At home they said I should come here because they didn't want me to go to the mountain."

Xolani Pikkie, a filmmaker who went through a Xhosa initiation ceremony 12 years ago, says the benefits are immense. "From a practical and health perspective I support it … I'd hate to have sex with a raincoat on," he says.

Complicating the scale-up in South Africa is communicating the fact that male circumcision – despite its health benefits – does not preclude condom use as there is still a risk of contracting HIV. Some argue that so important is the communication campaign that it should precede the rollout.

"It feels like we're losing the communication battle yet we haven't even started," says Pierre Brouard, deputy director of the University of Pretoria's Centre for the Study of AIDS.

And there is also a fear of publicising the service before systems are ready. "One could get long waiting lists and dissatisfaction," says Dr Sue Goldstein of the Soul City Institute for Health and Development Communications.

The rollout is due despite the vexed questions surrounding medical male circumcision. While initial fears were that the procedure gives men a false sense of security while hampering women from negotiating safe sex, research has shown little decrease in condom use or increase in risky behaviour. Clinical trials have also shown that it offers no direct protection to female partners.

Women themselves don't seem overly preoccupied with it. "It's not something I have thought about," says Lindiwe, a 26-year-old counsellor at Chris Hani Baragwanath Hospital. But Lisa Vetten, a researcher and policy analyst at the Tshwaranang Legal Advocacy Centre to End Violence Against Women, says the efficacy of male circumcision should provide incentive to continue development of a microbicide and other interventions that protect women directly. The rollout needs to be accompanied by a campaign "to make it clear that just because a man is circumcised doesn't mean he's safe," she said.

Part of the argument put forward by critics is that conditions prevailing in a medical trial do not provide a conclusive indication of the social dynamics that accompany male circumcision in the real world. This includes the failure to consider meanings associated with sexuality and gender sensitivity.

"The other area we are struggling with in South Africa is the tension between medical circumcision and traditional circumcision," Brouard points out. About 40 men died in the winter of 2010 in traditional initiation practices, which often do not remove the entire foreskin, thereby offering little or no protection from HIV. The question is how to convince the many men who are traditionally circumcised that they probably do not have the full protection that the procedure offers against the virus.

Researchers estimate that expanding circumcision services to 80 per cent of adult and newborn males in southern Africa would save $20.2 billion in HIV-related health costs between 2009 and 2025.

The Treatment Action Campaign is among those that support medical male circumcision.

"Pitting prevention against treatment is unhelpful," says TAC researcher Catherine Tomlinson. "We are seeing increasing evidence that antiretroviral therapy is an important prevention tool and that the dichotomy between prevention and treatment is actually false."

Dirk Taljaard, manager of Orange Farm's Bophelo Pele Circumcision Centre, estimates that South Africa needs to rapidly circumcise the "backlog" of some eight million men before scaling down to concentrate on the newly born.

While Dr Motsoaledi says each province is free to design its own treatment programme, he would rather voluntary medical male circumcision is not incorporated into the existing health system but is a stand-alone project. "I wouldn't like it to be part of every day hospital work ... integration would overwhelm normal hospital activities," he says.

Taljaard agrees. "We need sites where we can do a high volume of men in a very short space of time but also make sure that the quality is fine and that the aesthetics and safety measure up," he says.

WHO guidelines suggest that a scale-up should not be contemplated if the health system cannot be matched up with trained health personnel and other resources. But Professor Geoff Setswe, co-chair of the South African National AIDS Council's technical subcommittee on research, monitoring and evaluation, says the same argument was used against the introduction of antiretroviral drugs, yet South Africa now has the largest treatment programme in the world. "With male circumcision, it's an operation that – unlike antiretroviral treatment – is done once and is not to be repeated," he says.

Given the scale of the AIDS epidemic in South Africa, there is no time to waste, says Taljaard. "We need to be able to do it for two or three years and then we'll stop, it will be done," he says.

Originally published as "Men urged to snip in fresh assault on AIDS" in The New Age *on 23 September 2010.*

Orange Farm blazes the trail

Wilson Johwa

Outside of Johannesburg, a clinic in Orange Farm is leading the way for the drive to offer medical male circumcision as an HIV-prevention method.

On a typical day, but especially on Saturday mornings and over the school holidays, the Bophelo Pele project at Orange Farm teems mainly with boys barely out of their teens. The centre circumcised some 110 men a day in the winter of 2010 – about twice its normal average.

Located just outside Johannesburg, near Soweto, Bophelo Pele has also become a pilot site for what would be a workable model in a national medical male circumcision campaign. Among those queuing for the procedure are boys who would otherwise have gone to the bush for traditional initiation rites, but are either too far from their rural homes or are turned off by the reported deaths at circumcision schools in parts of the Eastern Cape. "I would have gone to the mountain because my brother went there last year," says 15-year-old Clinton Sebako whose traditional home is in the North West.

But others are here for different reasons, such as the belief that the procedure improves sexual performance, or merely for its social value rooted in tradition. "At home they said I should come here and not go to the mountains," says Molefe Dlamini. His friend Mzwakhe Mthembu cuts in: "If you have not been circumcised, you do sex a short time, not long," he says.

Twenty-year-old Sibusiso Zwane says he did it for health reasons. "I just did it to prevent diseases." Orange Farm was the location of one of three sites for clinical trials, which in 2005 concluded that male circumcision is 60 per cent effective against HIV. The other two sites were in Uganda and Kenya, showing similar results.

From 2008, Bophelo Pele offered circumcision to males from the area, partly to test the uptake of the procedure as a public health tool. Over 20 000 men were circumcised within an 18-month period.

"We think we are getting very close to the saturation point in Orange Farm where we have circumcised most of the eligible men – or at least the kind of percentage we can hope for," says Dirk Taljaard, manager of the project.

With funding from the President's Emergency Plan for AIDS Relief (PEPFAR), now just about anybody from anywhere can come for a circumcision. "It's a one-day procedure. You do the counselling and the testing and everything on the same day. You do all of that in the morning and in the afternoon you can circumcise," says Taljaard.

The centre has developed a single-use kit that costs R140 but the service is offered free of charge – a factor that has quite likely contributed to the strong interest in the procedure.

While the project kept a low profile for fear of being shut down during the controversial tenure of former Health Minister Manto Tshabalala-Msimang, it now offers lessons of what to expect in the proposed scale-up. For example, Taljaard says one surprise has been that about 42 per cent of men claiming to be circumcised were only partially circumcised – the foreskin having been only partially removed, most commonly in a traditional procedure.

The Farm has developed a "conveyor belt" model of mass circumcisions, due to be used in mass campaigns in neighbouring countries. "The model we have built in Orange Farm is based on multiple beds where a surgeon moves from one bed to the next, just performing the part of the operation that he needs to do," Taljaard says. Support staff prepare patients and also wrap up after an operation, allowing each of the project's three doctors to do eight to 10 procedures an hour.

But this is still not fast enough, as arresting the HIV tide requires the greatest number of men to be circumcised in the shortest possible time, says Taljaard. In countries such as Kenya and Botswana, nurses and other health personnel have been trained to perform circumcisions, a model that may be hard to replicate locally due to a shortage of health personnel.

Despite medical male circumcision being a scientifically contested procedure, Taljaard says the data on it has been among the most studied. "We do get a lot of criticism from people saying it is mutilation or that we are like a factory – you can say that if you're living in a country where HIV prevalence is 2 per cent. But if you live in Africa where HIV prevalence is 24 per cent, you cannot brush it off like that," he says.

Originally published as "Orange Farm leads new fight against HIV" in The New Age *on 23 September 2010.*

Not just (fore)skin deep

Wilson Johwa

Male circumcision is commonly referred to as a simple snip, but the reality is that there are many ways to skin the proverbial cat. People's motivations for electing the procedure can be equally varied. Wilson Johwa reviews the methods and reasons behind male circumcision.

Circumcisions are performed among men of various age groups, from newborns to over-forties, for religious, cultural or social reasons.

Men may also elect to do the procedure on purely medical grounds. Advantages of circumcision include reduced risk of penile cancer, STIs (notably syphilis), HPV, fewer urinary tract infections and an up to 60 per cent risk reduction of HIV infection. This is commonly attributed to the fact that the softer tissue on the foreskin is considerably more susceptible to pathogens, including the HI virus.

Medical male circumcision is also recommended for premature ejaculation, as well as for correcting a condition called phimosis, which is characterised by a tight foreskin that does not easily retract. For female partners, circumcision reduces the risk of cervical cancer and chlamydia. Improved hygiene is also frequently cited as a reason for removing the foreskin.

The evidence that medical male circumcision reduces the chances of contracting HIV by up to 60 per cent has resulted in countries within the southern African region embarking on a major scale-up of the procedure.

With so many people set to go through the procedure, safety concerns have become paramount. This requires for the procedure to be standardised.

Currently there are three common surgical methods for medical male circumcision. While non-surgical options exist, mostly consisting of clamps or rings, they have been associated with more complications. In particular, a Malaysian device known as the Tara KLamp, used by the KwaZulu-Natal provincial health department, has drawn criticism over its safety.

Surgical techniques range from the forceps-guided method found in low-tech and low-cost environments like an outlying clinic, to the dorsal slit and the sleeve methods – both of which require more surgical skill, but are fairly routine in hospitals worldwide.

The forceps-guided snip

This method is most common among the three surgical techniques recommended by the World Health Organization. It has a reputation for being quick and inexpensive, making it ideal for clinics – the main outlets for the planned scale-up in South Africa.

After a local anaesthetic has been administered, the foreskin is pulled forward and forceps are attached to the part protruding beyond the head of the penis. Using the forceps as a guide, the excess foreskin is then cut off like a ring through both layers at the same time.

The forceps-guided method can be learned by surgical assistants but the cosmetic effect may be less satisfactory. Its critics say it does not necessarily result in a straight line, while bleeding may be more profuse, requiring more stitches.

But Dr Dino Rech, co-director of the Centre for HIV and AIDS Prevention Studies (CHAPS), the organisation that heads up the MMC facility at Orange Farm, differs. "The cosmetic effect is different but it has nothing to do with a straight line or additional bleeding. It has more to do with the amount of mucosa [excess tissue] left behind, which some people do not like," he says.

The dorsal slit

With the dorsal-slit method, the foreskin is again pulled forward but instead of cutting across the protruding skin, an incision is made into the foreskin up to the glans (head). The excess foreskin is then trimmed away by cutting around from the end of the slit. This method is often recommended for people with phimosis.

"It is more likely to be used by a surgeon in a private hospital than a GP," says Dr Sello Mashamaite of Zuzimpilo Clinic in downtown Johannesburg.

The sleeve method

The best cosmetic result may be obtained from the sleeve method, although it does require more surgical skill and leaves more room for error. With this method, the foreskin is not pulled forward. Instead two separate cuts are made right around the penis – one towards the base and the other closer to the glans, forming a sleeve or tube of now loose foreskin around the shaft. This excess foreskin is then removed and the remaining skin is sutured together.

Dr Rech says Swaziland, presently in the middle of an accelerated scale-up of voluntary male circumcision, is moving from the sleeve method to incorporate the forceps-guided technique. "They are doing both at the moment."

Traditional techniques

Traditional practitioners use a free-hand approach, sometimes called the finger-guided method which, according to Dr Mashamaite is not standardised. "The problem is that it is not scientific, it hasn't been reviewed," he says.

Johannesburg doctor, Dr Moshe Singer, who is also a Jewish rabbi, uses the traditional Jewish technique where the foreskin is pulled out in front of the glans. Much like a cigar guillotine, a metal shield with a slot in it is slid over the foreskin immediately in front of the glans and then a scalpel is run across the face of the shield to remove the foreskin.

"It's an accepted regular method," he says. Dr Singer uses the same method for newborns and adults, including Jewish and non-Jewish men. "It gives a very clean, nice result; one can do it under local anaesthetic and the pain is surprisingly low."

A Jewish ritual circumcision is also called a Bris and, like other traditional methods of circumcision, it precludes the use of clamps.

Clamps

Circumcision devices or clamps pose a new challenge for local health authorities as they are not regulated and thus open to be used in an unmonitored fashion.

KwaZulu-Natal has led the scale-up of medical male circumcision in South Africa, with over 5 000 procedures having been done since the programme started in April 2010. However, use of the Tara KLamp has drawn unwanted publicity to the provincial health department, amid plans to circumcise 2.5 million men over the next five years. The Tara KLamp works by means of locking plastic arms that cut blood supply from the foreskin, causing it – along with the clamp – to fall off after a week. The Treatment Action Campaign and the Southern African HIV Clinicians Society insist that this causes more pain and that in some instances the clamp does not fall off, forcing the patient to have it surgically removed.

A small trial of young men at Orange Farm, a township near Soweto, found that those circumcised with the Tara KLamp were far more likely to report bleeding and swelling than those circumcised with forceps. Dr Rech says the Tara KLamp also needs to be compared to other available devices such as the ShangRing, which has had good results in China and in initial trials in Kenya. "Once this has been done and an independent assessment concluded, and if the Tara KLamp is then found to be safe and preferable, I will have no issues with its use," he says.

The ShangRing is named after its inventor, Jian-Zhong Shang, and consists of two concentric plastic rings that sandwich the foreskin, allowing it to be cut away without suturing and with minimal bleeding.

Marketers of the Tara KLamp, including the KwaZulu-Natal health department, say it is cost effective as it does not require a surgeon, only a trained male nurse. The province's health minister Sibongiseni Dhlomo said participants are able to choose between the clamp and the forceps-guided method. His spokesman Chris Maxon says an evaluation report would soon be released on the efficacy of the clamp to date. "The Minister has also set up a task team to look into the implementation so as to guide policy and practice," he says.

Despite the variety of methods for medical male circumcision, the practice is among a wide array of interventions adopted by the South African government in its bid to curb HIV infection. Yet controversy over use of the Tara KLamp is likely to cloud South Africa's scale-up of male circumcision. Despite health concerns, Health Minister Dr Aaron Motsoaledi ruled out its removal from the market. "We're not married to any particular one clamp," he says, blaming a gap in the regulations, which leaves medical gadgets unregulated.

However, this is expected to change when the Health Department replaces the Medicines Control Council with a new body, the South African Health Products Regulatory Authority, which will regulate medical gadgets in addition to medicines. "It will definitely be through an Act of Parliament," he says.

Blog: Getting in gear

Wilson Johwa

Implementing a medical male circumcision policy will require careful negotiation of social and behavioural issues.

It is now too late for my 14-year-old son to be circumcised – at least that's what he seems to think. In his view, the procedure should have been done when he was younger and less aware of the pain. "It's embarrassing," he says, refusing to buy into the argument that in 1995 when he was born, the impact of HIV was only just unfolding and there would have been no need for him to be circumcised.

Within medical circles in much of Africa there is now a strong recognition that male circumcision lowers the risk of HIV transmission. The sooner the procedure is performed on a male, the better. But infant circumcision still has its fair share of sceptics, including a team of Australian researchers whose work was published in a recent issue of the *Annals of Family Medicine*. They argue that not enough work has been done on the psychological impact of male circumcision, especially the fact that it could potentially cause anger, feelings of incompleteness, hurt, or being violated.

The review's lead author, Dr Caryn Perera of the Australasian College of Surgeons, said the risk of major complications ranged from 2 per cent to 10 per cent. "These may be considered unacceptable for an elective procedure," she told *HealthDay News*.

However, in a country like South Africa where HIV-related complications are the major cause of death, these figures are likely to be seen as an unfortunate but unavoidable consequence of a potentially life-saving procedure.

Yet the psychological and social effects of medical male circumcision are no idle consideration, especially for communities that traditionally do not circumcise either for religious or cultural reasons. Such unchartered waters may account for the delay in the government rolling out a male circumcision strategy, despite talk that circumcision is the next frontier in the fight against the AIDS pandemic.

But not everyone is taken in. Pierre Brouard, deputy director at the University of Pretoria's Centre for the Study of AIDS, concedes that male circumcision as an HIV-prevention strategy comes with a number of challenges.

Messaging around circumcision needs to be approached cautiously since the procedure only offers partial protection, making condoms a necessity to fully avoid sexually transmitted infections. Of course pregnancy is an entirely different matter and circumcision will not offer any contraceptive benefits. This also needs to be highlighted.

Brouard says, "Communities need to be advised and prepared for circumcision and there are concerns that in a highly gendered epidemic male circumcision could play into patriarchal attitudes towards women."

A clinical psychologist, Brouard feels that the psychological issues are not to be taken lightly.

Male circumcision may play into traditional ideas of what it means to be a man – or rather a certain idea of a man who needs to "prove" his masculinity, and complete his journey to full male adulthood.

But Brouard does not believe that psychological issues will discourage MMC's adoption on a mass scale. Instead, he says male circumcision is already well established in many communities in South Africa.

All this makes male circumcision as a prevention strategy a work in progress, particularly given concern that biomedical interventions of this nature are rarely accompanied by research on the wider social impact of the proposed action.

The World Health Organization, together with UNAIDS, have backed the evidence that male circumcision provides up to 60 per cent protection against HIV. In March 2007, they finalised recommendations encouraging countries with a high HIV prevalence and low levels of male circumcision to scale-up on the procedure. But at this stage there are no governmental guidelines on medical male circumcision, which is still a matter of individual choice and a sector dominated mainly by non-governmental projects, such as Zuzimpilo, which operates in downtown Johannesburg.

In March 2010, Health Minister Aaron Motsoaledi announced the country's largest-ever testing and counselling campaign with a price tag of R1.4 billion. It would consume some 2.5 billion male condoms over the following year and see 15 million tested for HIV by 2011.

At the official level, male circumcision is a strategy that will come with much preparation. "Gearing up health systems to address the demand will take time, resources and planning," says Brouard.

The area of traditional circumcision poses another set of challenges. Many circumcisions that were performed traditionally do not involve removal of the entire foreskin, thus not offering the same protection as the medical procedure.

"Cultural guardians may also be reluctant to have their traditions in any way interfered with," says Brouard.

Originally published on journAIDS.org *on 21 April 2010.*

Blog: Debating manhood at Orange Farm

Wilson Johwa

Wilson Johwa speaks to the men waiting to get "the snip" at Orange Farm's circumcision centre.

At Orange Farm, a township outside Johannesburg, boys barely out of their teens and full-grown men sit together in a queue as they wait to be circumcised. Had I not arrived at 9 am to find a fully formed queue of men and boys, I would not have believed that this winter an average of just over 100 men and adolescents are circumcised here every day. This is twice the average number recorded per day in summer.

While a few boys mill around the entrance, about eight are already in a communal counselling room, prior to seeing counsellors individually. The nurses are casually preparing the main surgery room, which has seven beds. They unwrap circumcision packs – each costing R140 and packed specially for the centre.

The other surgery, with two beds, is upstairs and is often used for older participants who require a little more privacy. The manager of the centre, Daniel Shabangu, tells me that the oldest participant they ever had was 68 years old. "He came with his son and we circumcised them together," Shabangu says.

Today, most of the participants are young, barely out of their teens. Some have come a long way, as far afield as Tembisa. They all mention a desire to prevent HIV and other sexually transmitted infections. Clearly they are well counselled. George seems more honest, confessing to having had "drop" – a sexually transmitted infection.

Someone says it is better to do it here than in the mountains.

I get a nod when I ask about whether enhanced sexual pleasure is among the reasons they are here. But Themba, a 24-year-old I catch on the steps on his way to the surgery upstairs, is the most forthcoming on this point. "It relaxes after circumcision, and may get bigger," he says, in all seriousness.

Dirk Taljaard, co-founder of the centre, had told me that it appears many men come because deep down they had always wanted to be circumcised, perhaps to complete the transformation into what they believe a man has to be. I wonder if the desire for enhanced sexual performance is what drives many men to circumcise.

It is apparent that the large numbers at Orange Farm are due to any one or all of these reasons, including that there is no fee for the procedure. My visit is during school holidays, and winter is not yet over. The belief that it is better to do it in winter seems to survive. But Shabangu dismisses the assertion that healing is better in winter, saying this is not borne by evidence.

Being at Orange Farm on a cold morning in winter left me with mixed feelings and a strong appreciation of just how complex male circumcision is. Each man is here on his own free will. Each is here for his own reason, informed by myth or reality. It is hard to fathom what male circumcision actually means to everybody aside from offering protection against HIV and STIs.

Originally published on journAIDS.org *on 12 August 2010.*

Contributors

Contributors

Willemien Brümmer was born in Cape Town in 1974, the daughter of a storyteller-mathematician and a mother who works in the disability field. After completing honours degrees in Journalism and Drama at Stellenbosch University, she earned a master's degree in Creative Writing (cum laude) at the University of Cape Town. Her first book is a collection of short stories, *Die dag toe ek my hare losgemaak het* (Human & Rousseau, 2008). Brümmer started working as a journalist in 1999. She worked as *Die Burger's* medical reporter with a special interest in HIV and was the writer of *Oop Kaarte*, the newspaper's profiles. After her time at *Die Burger*, she was specialist reporter at the now defunct magazine *INSIG*, and then started working for *By*, an in-depth features supplement, which appears with *Die Burger*, *Beeld* and *Volksblad*. She is currently the Rykie van Reenen Fellow at the University of Stellenbosch, where she teaches News and Feature Writing to the BPhil class of 2012. She has won many awards – among them a Mondi for Feature Writing and a Vodacom Journalist of the Year, also in the Features category. In 2012 she was awarded two ATKV-Mediaveertjies in the categories Best Profile and Best Arts Journalism.

Thabisile Dlamini, at age 25, boasts a list of achievements. In 2007, as a second-year Media and Journalism student at Boston Media College, Dlamini already had her byline in the national youth magazine *UNCUT*. In 2008 she produced radio content for loveLife. The talk shows were broadcast in all official languages on SABC and smaller community radio stations. In 2009 she moved into digital media and, with a "new media" consultant from New York, produced a "first" in South Africa – a youth mobile social network dedicated to social change, *www.mymsta.mobi*. For Dlamini, 2011 marked a career change and she took up a leading role in the local musical *My Richest Yard* at the South African State Theatre during the Rain of Art festival. Dlamini is currently a voice-over artist in the loveLife radio drama *Foxy Chix*, broadcast on Ukhozi fm. Seeking to broaden her knowledge and skills, she is also studying music with

UNISA and taking private acting lessons. Dlamini is currently working on a motivational book on human dignity, as well as a novel.

Nardus Engelbrecht is a photographer living in Cape Town. His work has been published in various newspapers, magazines and books. He started freelancing in 2008 when he moved from Johannesburg to Cape Town. In Johannesburg he worked as a press photographer for Media24.

Wilson Johwa is a journalist with *Business Day* newspaper in Johannesburg. He holds a BA (Hons) in Journalism and Media Studies from the University of the Witwatersrand and has 14 years' media experience, working mainly in Zimbabwe and South Africa.

Lungi Langa is a young, aspiring health journalist who has worked for the non-profit health news agency, health-e. During her time at health-e, she wrote on a variety of issues ranging from HIV, TB and the N1H1 flu pandemic to the doctors' strike. She completed her Journalism Diploma at the Durban University of Technology in KwaZulu-Natal in 2006. Langa served as a media intern at Art for Humanity (AFH), a non-profit organisation specialising in HIV and women and children's rights. In her writing she strives to capture the human aspect of people's stories by portraying their day-to-day struggles, challenges and triumphs as they face the prejudice and stigma frequently associated with illness. By giving them a face, she hopes to contribute to eradicating a mindset that so often reduces people to mere "statistics".

Melissa Meyer coordinates the HIV & AIDS Media Project, a partnership between the Wits Journalism Programme and the Anova Health Institute. Soon after qualifying as a journalist (University of Johannesburg), she developed a keen interest in the political management of the HIV epidemic, pursuing it with an MA in Political Studies (UJ). In 2009 she went on to co-author a book on the subject with Pieter Fourie, titled *The Politics of AIDS Denialism: South Africa's failure to respond* (Ashgate). Meyer is passionate about tailoring effective and audience-appropriate communication, and in 2010 extended this interest to the field of visual communication with a qualification in Graphic Design (AAA). As coordinator of the project, she delivers regular commentary on the media's engagement with HIV and, through media training and journalism support, continues to work towards facilitating communication that is healthy.

Lebohang Mashiloane is a 30-year-old documentary photographer based in Johannesburg. He studied Fine Art photography at the Vaal University of Technology and later Advanced Photojournalism and Documentary at the MarketPhoto Workshop. He was also selected for Digital Journalism at the International Institute for Journalism in Berlin, Germany, in 2006. Mashiloane previously worked as a photojournalist at *The Star* and later *The Times* in Johannesburg. His work has been showcased in the Bamako Biennale in Mali, a premium African Photography Festival, and later toured to different countries as part of the festival's collective exhibition. He is currently starting his own multimedia company, See.mo Media.

Helen Struthers is co-founder and co-director of the HIV & AIDS Media Project, a partnership between the Wits Journalism Programme and the Anova Health Institute. Since 2002 she has led a large multi-disciplinary HIV research and support programme primarily funded by USAID. She holds an MBA (Wits) and MSc in Applied Mathematics (Wits). Struthers has published extensively on the medical and social aspects of HIV. She is currently reading for her PhD, pursuing her enduring research interest in masculinity and HIV, in particular men who have sex with men.

Mthetho C Tshemese is a registered clinical psychologist, Clinton Democracy Fellow, public commentator and social entrepreneur. His research interests include masculinity, *ulwaluko* (traditional male circumcision), suicide, youth culture and music. Tshemese is currently with the Mental Health Unit at the Nelson Mandela Academic Hospital Mthatha, in the Eastern Cape. He is working on his PhD, focusing on *ulwaluko* and masculinity in the Eastern Cape.

Pieter van Zyl has been a journalist for almost 10 years. After completing his studies in literature at the University of NorthWest in Potchefstroom, he moved to Johannesburg where he began working as a crime reporter for the daily Afrikaans newspaper *Die Beeld*. The following year, 2000, he received the Willem Wepener trophy for Most Promising Young Reporter. In 2001 Van Zyl began working for *Die Burger* in Port Elizabeth, where he was a senior writer, weekend news editor and arts and entertainment editor. In 2004 he moved to Cape Town to start working on the editorial staff of one of the biggest magazines in South Africa – *Huisgenoot* (Afrikaans) and *YOU* (English). There, Van Zyl reports on anything from sports stars to celebrity weddings, human tragedy, inspirational real-life events and political issues. Van Zyl also seeks to encourage others by writing about how he has risen above his own mental health challenges. In 2007 he was awarded the Rosalynn Fellowship for Mental Health Journalism in Atlanta, Georgia, USA.